Vital Sensation Manual

UNIT TWO:
LEVELS

**Based on
The Sensation Method
& Classical Homeopathy**

Written
by
Melissa Burch, CCH, & Susana Aikin, CCH

Edited by Ingrid Dankmeyer, Didi Pershouse and Sharon Willis

Cover Design by Chetana Deorah

Text Design by Janet Innes and George Papargyris

Published by
Inner Health, Inc.
175 Harvey St., #13
Cambridge, MA 02140
(617) 491-3374
melissa@innerhealth.us
www.innerhealth.us

© 2011, Inner Health, Inc.

TABLE OF CONTENTS

A. INTRODUCTION

Levels of experience are one of the most important guiding tools in the process of casetaking. In the journey of casetaking, it gives us the routes as to where we are and how to proceed further.

Dr. Rajan Sankaran
Bombay 2003

When homeopaths take a case, they initiate a journey of discovery that will run through all the layers of the patient's human experience in search for the necessary information that will lead to the selection of a curative remedy. Through this journey the homeopath will pursue deeper and deeper levels of the patient's state in order to grasp the essence of disharmony and match it with a similar substance. This vertical descent into the patient's consciousness can be a difficult process that has never been properly mapped. The theory of levels is an attempt to map the layers of human experience in order to facilitate the homeopathic journey.

The idea of levels is not new. Already Hahnemann and Kent talked about the spiritual and anatomical levels of man. Hahnemann distinguished five levels: the Organism, the Organic Vital Force, the Vital Force, the Dynamis and the Vital Principle, which is the highest level. Kent talked about the Will (analogous to the Vital Principle), the Intellect (Dynamis), the Fluids (Vital Force), Internal Organs (Organic Vital Force) and finally External Organs (Organism). The need for establishing levels also arose in them as a means to better locate disharmony in the structure of the human being and select an appropriate homeopathic substance.

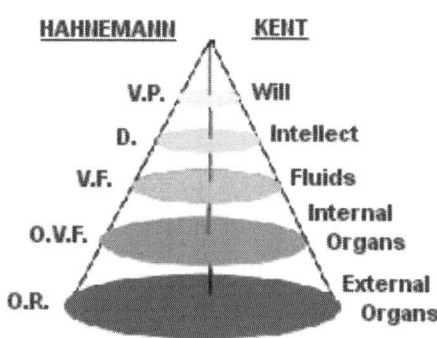

Diagram of the Cone and Levels in Man

Diagram from "Samuel Hahnemann Organon of Medicine with explanations by Joseph Reaves" (Homoeopress Limited 1994)

Recently, Sankaran has also come up with another system of levels to help map the different levels of human consciousness. In his system, there are seven levels starting with: 1. Name, 2. Fact, 3. Emotion, 4. Delusion, 5. Sensation, 6. Energy, and 7. Seventh level.

This scheme is based on the different depths of human experience and perception. A person standing in front of a mountain might perceive just a name (i.e. Everest), or the facts related to that mountain (i.e. tallest mountain in the world, first climbed to the summit in May 1953), or might experience the mountain primarily as an emotional experience where he might feel overwhelmed by its beauty or magnificence. The person can also experience the mountain at the level of Delusion, where they would see it as an overpowering, insurmountable obstacle; or even at the level of Sensation where they would feel lightness and floating. At the level of Energy, they might feel oneness with the mountain, and finally at level 7 they would plunge into pure consciousness and silence.

The objective of the casetaking journey is to find the Vital Sensation through the descent into deeper levels. The Vital Sensation can be detected at any level, although eventually needs to be confirmed at all levels. This system of levels based on degrees of perception and consciousness can be very useful to the homeopath in casetaking as a map in which to track the disease and disharmony in the patient. As the homeopath pursues the Chief Complaint in the case, the patient will move through the levels giving the practitioner the possibility to access deeper levels of information not obscured by compensation or personal interpretation.

Homeopathy can be practiced at any of these different levels with successful prescriptions. It can be practiced at the pathological level (level of Name), for example giving Sabal Serrulata for enlarged prostate, or Carduus Marianus for an enlarged liver. Homeopaths can practice homeopathy at the level of Fact (level 2), giving Bryonia to a patient, who complains of chest pain worse from movement. They can also practice at the level of Emotion (level 3) and give Ignatia Amara for a patient who has been disappointed in love, or give Stramonium for a child who has fear of the dark. Homeopathy can also be practiced at the level of Delusion (level 4), and a patient can be prescribed Mercury because she feels surrounded by enemy. Many of the prescriptions given at these different levels can be very good. However, delving into deeper levels will definitely increase the homeopath's success rates since there are more layers to confirm the homeopath's perception of what needs to be cured and what is the best similimum for the case.

In the past homeopaths have been working with some of these levels: the old masters were geniuses at prescribing at the first two levels (Name and Fact), and Kent already pointed at the emotional level of remedies (i.e. the suppressed anger of Staphysagria). Later, homeopathic prescriptions largely based on delusions became a widespread practice after the work of George Vithoulkas, Jan Scholten and that of Sankaran himself. Through further investigation Sankaran, when studying plant remedies, came up with the concept of the level of Sensation. Before that homeopaths knew that the kingdom of plants was characterized by sensitivity, in contrast with structure for minerals and survival for animals.

Sankaran decided to extract common rubrics specific to plant families and discovered strong similar sensations running through families of plants. This discovery opened up sensation as a basic experiential concept in which to categorize raw feelings and perceptions common to human beings and homeopathic substances. Sankaran realized that once patients reached this level of Sensation, they were able to bypass the rational mind and give direct uncompensated information to the homeopath. He saw it was at this level that the homeopath could best determine the Vital Sensation, as well as the kingdom and the miasm of the case. In further explorations he realized that all patients will speak about sensations in relation to their Chief Complaint and that the level of Sensation exists in all kingdoms. The discovery of the level of Energy and the 7th level followed suit.

In the past the homeopath was looking at a collection of symptoms, mental states or delusions by connecting the various elements and then would come to an understanding of the totality. Now the homeopath can perceive and use these levels to understand both patients and remedies, which is far beyond the duality of mind and the body. At this level, where mind and body intersect, lies the Vital Sensation, which when properly explored reveals the direct connection between the patient's state and the energy pattern of the remedy. This technique of casetaking, which relentlessly probes the Chief Complaint, becomes the vehicle that will take us accurately through the different levels. The final objective is to reach an understanding of the Vital Sensation at all levels and in particular at the level of Sensation that will reveal the full totality of the case.

It is better for homeopaths not to work out of one level but to have constant access to all the levels of the case. The homeopath can confirm the prescription found through this method by making sure that the strange, rare and peculiar symptoms also fall within the scope of the remedy. Most times this confirmation is made by checking the original provings. The main benefit of the system of levels is to offer access to multiple levels, wherein the homeopath can find the Vital Sensation and confirm it throughout the case.

B. PHILOSOPHY OF LEVELS

Defining levels is an exercise in mapping the spectrum of consciousness in the being we intend to heal. Disease is a manifestation of disharmony at different levels of consciousness. Disease and disharmony can be seen as the usurpation of consciousness by a different energy which is foreign to the organism. When the energy of a different being or substance takes over our consciousness we become diseased. When we are exposed to the mirroring effect of a similimum, we become conscious of our fixation and release it. For example, when we are infected by a bacterium or virus, its intention is not to harm us but to survive. Syphilis, for instance, is the consciousness in the body of the syphilitic bacteria, Treponema pallidum. The body tries to resist the bacteria, keep it localized, as a means to keep its own identity untouched by isolating it through the production of local symptoms. In the process tissue might be destroyed and pathology ensues. As the disease advances, the new invading agent gains progressive hold over the host's consciousness. Our deepest deranged states of mind, the mental diseases, would then be a moment in which the foreign entity has gained complete consciousness of the human being. At that point, we don't recognize the patient's behavior anymore, and we call them insane.

In this sense, a Hyoscyamus patient will suddenly expose herself in public. A Veratrum album person will be preaching loudly about the apocalypse. The right remedy reveals the unhealthy state of being to our inner consciousness and gives relief. In a diseased state we are compelled to follow the purpose of the other being's existence. In a state of health, we are free to follow the purpose of our own existence. For example, if a patient needs Lac Lioninum and is cured, the person does not become a better lion but a healthy human being. The realization of the disease state by homeopathy, meditation or other means helps us release the consciousness of the foreign entity and eventually reach the fullness of human potential.

The Seventh level is the beginning from which the level of Energy is created, which imprints the Sensation level, which then creates the Delusion level, which then generates the Emotion level, and which then brings Fact and Name. Levels of consciousness arise from each other. All levels are interconnected, and each level is created from the immediate deeper level. Within each level there is also a spectrum of consciousness that ranges from the upper level to the lower level. For example, at the level of Emotion, expressions of Name, Fact, Delusion, Sensation, Energy and 7th level are also present. Disease permeates all levels following the same direction from 7th level down to all other levels, and cure affects all the levels affected by the disease, usually in the opposite direction level 1, Name, to 7th level (Herring's Law).

The seven levels can be used to map different aspects related to Homeopathy.

For example, the levels of prescription in Homeopathy:

Level 1   Pathological
Level 2   Symptomatic

Level 3   Emotional
Level 4   Delusional
Level 5   Sensational
Level 6   Energy based

The patient experiences his problems both physically and mentally at different levels.

For example, the levels of physical symptoms:

Level 1   Diagnosis Pathology
Level 2   Local symptoms, location-sensation-modality
Level 3   Concomitants, general effects of complaint
Level 4   NEI (Neuro-Endocrino-Immunological)
           cravings, sleep, generals, modalities
Level 5   General sensations and affections
Level 6   General movements and patterns

For example, the levels of sensitivity:

Level 1   Not sensitive
Level 2   Locally sensitive
Level 3   Sensitive in feelings
Level 4   Sensitive in mind
Level 5   Sensitive in most basic issues
Level 6   Universal and intense sensitivity

For example, the levels and the nervous system:

Level 1   Hypothalamic (autonomic)
Level 2   Intellect
Level 3   Emotion
Level 4   Imagination
Level 5   Sensitivity
Level 6   Vitality
Level 7   Consciousness

It is also possible to consider the relationship between human age and the seven levels. Conception takes place at the 7th level and the ensuing incarnation of the child occurs at the Energy level, where also infancy develops. Childhood is lived at the level of Delusion, young adulthood is at the level of Emotion, and as we age we move more into Facts and finally Name. Children want to listen to stories and watch movies full of imagination; as they become adults they get into melodramas, then as people age they move into news, weather and stock prices; finally in the older stages, people are happy just to remember names of people. As adults there is a tendency to deal with reality at the intellectual level (level of Fact) and eventually narrow down to the level of Name.

Level 1   Senility
Level 2   Old age

Level 3   Middle age
Level 4   Teenage
Level 5   Childhood
Level 6   Infancy
Level 7   Conception and Death

The same spectrum of consciousness also applies to other areas of human expression. There are levels in entertainment, communication, art, music or any other human experience. Art can simply depict fact, like a detailed portrait of a king on his throne; it can also express emotion, like "Mona Lisa," or imagination, such as Salvador Dali's "Persistence of Memory." There is also art at the level of sensations and energy (i.e. Rothko and Mondrian). Similarly, music can also be at the level of Facts (commercial jingle) or emotions (Blues), delusions (Pink Floyd), sensations (Beethoven), and energy (African drums, Tibetan bells).

C. THE SEVEN LEVELS

Level 1: Name

Here the patient experiences and identifies with the pathological diagnosis of the situation. For example, they talk about their problem as having prostate enlargement, migraines, arthritis, depression, schizophrenia, etc.

Level 2: Fact

The patient describes the elements of reality of the situation. For instance, she will describe the symptoms of the pathology like pain in the knee. The patient qualifies the situation by describing sensations, location and modalities. For example, my headache is in the supraorbital region and only in the evening, and is made better by tight pressure; or my arthritis feels like a burning pain, which is made worse by motion.

This is mostly the level of keynote prescriptions, (i.e. an Arsenicum patient has burning pains relieved by heat). The emotions at this level or even the sensations are exclusively local. For example, when I get my migraines, I feel very irritable (emotion at the level of Fact). The concomitants would also be local at this level. For example, when I get my wheezing asthmatic attacks, I feel itching in the chin.

Level 3: Emotion

The patient describes feelings associated with the facts. She will describe emotions like anger, irritability, sadness, grief, joy, etc. At this level the emotions are felt but might not be specific to the complaint. They will explore and express their feelings about their situation. For example, I am struggling with my marriage and feel abandoned. In the concomitants at the level of Emotion, the homeopath can observe feelings that also affect the Chief Complaint. For instance, when the patient fights with her husband and gets angry, she gets a migraine.

Level 4: Delusion

The level of Delusion is characterized by powerful images. The emotions are felt intensely and are associated with a specific situation or scene. Delusion is an expression of the sensation in the human form. The patient projects pictures and scenes. For example, a patient, who feels obligated to take care of his community, sees himself as Atlas bearing the burden of the whole world on his shoulders.

So at this level the homeopath may make use of dreams, subconscious images, interests, hobbies and similar expressions from the patient. Most specifically dreams are often very expressive of delusions. Observing gestures, commonly used metaphors, precise images and imaginary situations is crucial at this level of casetaking. For example: My mother in law keeps fighting with me. She is troubling me and torturing me. It is like a tiger attacking me.

Level 5: Sensation

Beyond our imagination and its expression at the level of Delusion lies another realm that is completely non-human specific and belongs to the common ground of consciousness we share with plants, minerals and animals. The themes of survival (animal), structure (mineral) or sensitivity (plant) are revealed at this level. The level of sensation is where the patient expresses the raw experience of the situation. At this deeper level of Sensation the homeopath has a better chance of eliciting non-human specific language that expresses the Vital Sensation, which manifests throughout the whole case.

Sensation will be expressed as heat, cold, sharp, numbness, caught, pulled, contracted, expanded, brittle, pursued, tingling, and so forth. For example, a woman has pain in the sinus, which is extreme as if it would break off. It would be less painful to die. It is like a plate, inserting a plate. It could break apart. I wish it would burst my head. It was hurting on the whole plane, breaks into two, maybe it is going to do more damage inside me.

Even delusions are based on sensations. At the level of Sensation a lot of delusional language is expressed by the patient, however, the level of Sensation is more intangible, illogical and insane than a delusion. Delusions are construed as images or pictures that can be represented as novels or movies, but sensations cannot and are expressed in abstract forms of raw feelings. At the level of Sensation the duality between mind and body disappears and the Vital Sensation is most directly exposed. For example, a patient who is having a conflict says it is as if they are disturbing me, interrupting my life and my peace. This aversion to being disturbed (Violales plant family) is the main sensation. It is neither mental nor physical but this is common to both levels.

Emotions are felt very intensely at this level and with specific sensations. For example, the person has intense terror alternating with the sensation of numbness (Opium). Sensations are also well expressed in dreams. For example, in a case where the Vital Sensation is cut and stabbed, the patient could have a dream of being cut and hacked by soldiers (Bryonia). At this level the homeopath can confirm the kingdom of the case and the miasm.

Level 6: Energy

The energy pattern that arises from the Energy level manifests from within the person. It is a deep layer and beyond that there is silence. The way the patients embody energy patterns that arise from this level will determine the sensation and holds the fundamental energy, colors, shapes and movements of the specific kingdoms and remedies. The Energy level is a space that contains all possible shapes and forms that exist on the physical plane. Therefore, matter is structured at this level. The deepest possible cure happens at this level.

At this level it is difficult to observe the energy directly, but as the homeopath pursues the case deeper the patient's abstract gestures start unfolding and then it is possible to see energy patterns. The patient also expresses source language at this level. Source language is drawn from the collective consciousness, where the patient describes the attributes of the homeopathic substance they need. For example, a patient needing a plant remedy from the Conifer family talked about sticky, honey like, room temperature, not hot like lava, comes from a crack from a tube. The substance she was describing is sap from a tree. Terebinthina was prescribed successfully, which is turpentine, resinous exudates obtained from Coniferous trees.

Here at the Energy level the person is not experiencing the sensation but living it. Although Vital Sensation is easier to detect at the Sensation level, it originates at the Energy level. Very specific emotions and sensations are observed with energy patterns. Sometimes the homeopath can detect prominent energy patterns and relationships to specific substances from the source language the patient uses when describing their dreams. Every expression of a human being arises from the energy pattern (laughter, stride, tone of voice, etc.). Energy is observed by the way it moves through the patient. The force will have speed, sound, direction, color. Everything is expressing patterns all the time.

The Energy level is non-specific to kingdoms because remedies from different kingdoms can have similar energy patterns. For instance, three remedies belonging to plant, mineral and animal kingdoms can all have nearly the same energy patterns although they express it differently. This brings in the idea of correspondence. Some remedies in the plant kingdom correspond to others in the animal or mineral kingdom, and they share the similar energy pattern (e.g., analogous examples such as Mezereum and Mercury, Hyoscyamus and Naja, etc.). Similarly, two different patients, who require the same remedy, can have different delusions but cannot have different energy patterns.

The homeopath touches the Energy level, then the sensations become sharp and clear, and everything can open up in the case. The level of Energy is mostly unknown territory for most homeopaths at the present time.

Level 7: Silence, Consciousness

There is one more level which is beyond the Energy level, and that level is the screen on which all energy patterns can manifest. It is the basis of energy, just like Energy is the basis of Sensation; Sensation is the basis of Delusion; and Delusion is the basis of Emotion. In this sense the basis of all energy patterns is the level which is devoid of all energy patterns. It is a complete void and the canvas on which different things can happen. Some call it God or Consciousness. It is the deepest layer without sound, colour, light or movement, a complete blank. This is the level of the moment of death or of conception, the stage of coma, a stage of nothingness, an undifferentiated state. This is the connecting link that completes the cycle of all the levels.

D. USE OF LEVELS IN CASETAKING AND ANALYSIS

We are dealing with a world at various levels. We experience phenomena as identity, fact or emotion, and generally the consciousness or our experience stops there. Obviously this is only the very top layer of the experience. It is the tip of the iceberg and the remaining seven eighths of the mass lies below. This would not only be the sub-conscious mind, but even deeper uncharted levels. Mind itself is only the tip of the iceberg.

Dr. Rajan Sankaran, New York 2003

The system of levels works as a progression in the sense that there is a dynamic evolution from undifferentiated to more differentiated states. The pathological process also tends to follow this path, and can have the effect of disrupting the continuity of the different levels. Therefore, the mere act of connecting these levels together in the patient's consciousness through casetaking already initiates the healing process.

The map of levels is one of the most important guiding tools to show the homeopath where the patient is in the case and how to proceed further. The homeopath needs to pursue the Chief Complaint as the main path through the levels until the Vital Sensation is found. The homeopath needs to hold the patient at the level she is in before moving to another level. For example, the patient says this pulling makes me wild. The practitioner needs to understand everything about pulling (sensation at Fact level) before going to wild (possible Delusion level). Once the level is complete then the patient will move to another level.

It is important to be aware that the client will have signs and language of the level before and after the one she is in. For example, at the level of Delusion the homeopath will detect emotions and sensations. The language from other levels does not necessarily mean that the patient is at those other levels.

The homeopath will develop a perception of recognizing energy and energy patterns through casetaking and watching cases taken using this method. The patient's words that do not fit the description or are spoken after a long pause, gestures that are repeated or have an intensity (direction, speed and energy) or are out of context are possible indications of energy to pay attention to. When the homeopath observes the energy, gestures and words repeatedly, she will eventually realize an energy pattern called the Vital Sensation. The homeopath is not looking for specific words, but for the experience of the patient and the point where the energy lies in the case. Words along with gestures that hold energy are ultimately used to travel on this map and need to be identified and confirmed by the homeopath so that the Vital Sensation is recognized in the case.

The patient can follow various routes, for example: from Level 1, Name, to 2, Fact, to 3, Emotion, to 4, Delusion, to 5, Sensation, to 6, Energy, or sometimes from Level 2, Fact, to 5, Sensation, and then level 4, Delusion, then to level 3, Emotion, then level 4,

Delusion, and finally back to level 5, Sensation. As long as the patient is moving easily from one level to another, the homeopath follows along even if the patient is jumping from different levels and back again. Not all patients will flow easily from one level to another. Many cases will have a fixation at a specific level, in particular at the level of Emotion or Delusion. When the client gets stuck at a particular level, then a new approach is needed to take the patient to a deeper level. These techniques are called bypasses.

The following are examples of where patients become blocked at different levels:
The patient cannot move from level 2, Fact, to level 3, Emotion, when she is unable to describe her feelings after telling the various facts of her illness and after the practitioner asks: "What feelings are associated with it?"

The patient cannot move from level 3, Emotion, to level 4, Delusion, when she has difficulty giving images or a visual presentation after describing her emotions and after the practitioner asks: "How was it perceived?"

The patient cannot move from level 4, Delusion, to level 5, Sensation, when she is not able to give the sensation of the case, although she can give images.

The patient cannot move from Level 5, Sensation, to level 6, Energy, when she doesn't express the energy or any particular source language but describes her sensations well.

Level of Name

At the level of Name, the patient describes the pathology; for example, jaundice, cirrhosis or asthma. At this level it is rare to hear language pertaining to emotion, delusion, sensation or source when they describe the diagnosis of the complaints. Be aware of words or gestures that express energy that can lead the case further. Remember do not let go of the Chief Complaint. Tell the client to describe more about the problem. Ask: What is the diagnosis? How long has the problem existed? How often does the problem occur? These details will help in the treatment.

After the client has fully explained the pathology, ask the following questions in order to move to the next level:

> Describe more about your complaints.
> How does the complaint affect you?
> How does it affect your life?
> Which complaint bothers you the most?

Level of Fact

At the Level 2, Fact, the patient describes the various details of the problem. This is the level where the Chief Complaint is most times identified. The practitioner needs to understand it completely, have it qualified as much as possible and get all the peculiarities. Pay attention to any emotions, delusions and sensations. Observe the energy, the gestures and characteristic expressions that come up while describing the Chief Complaint. These observations will form the basis that will help to confirm the various aspects that come up later in the case. At the Fact level we have to understand the local sensation very precisely from the Chief Complaint and then see how this local sensation becomes general.

If there are no words with energy to unfold the case further or no local sensation, then ask the patient to describe more. If she describes more than one problem or goes to some other problems, note all the different complaints and ask which one is bothering her the most. If the patient gets lost with too many details, take her back to the Chief Complaint. If the patient diverts to emotional aspects, bring her back to the Chief Complaint again until the Fact level is exhausted.

The homeopath needs to ask what the problem is, have it qualified and then find out the peculiars. For example, it is a pain in the knee (what), worse with motion (qualified) and better from eating cucumbers (peculiar). At this level a local phenomenon can become general, when it is experienced in the same way in another location other than the Chief Complaint. The client may use the same sensation to describe their emotions or other physical phenomenon. For example, the patient says, "My knee gets stuck and feels blocked, and I'm feeling stuck at my job too." They can express through repeated gestures, or a gesture with intense energy. It may also be when they describe an experience very vividly or emphasize the same ideas over and over. Once the Fact level has been exhausted, if any word or image shows intense energy or is peculiar, follow the lead of the words or images into the next level.

Questions to ask at the level of Fact, which will lead to other levels:

> Describe it more.
> Which complaint bothers you the most?
> How does the complaint affect you?
> How does it affect your life?
> Describe more, not your complaints, but just the experience. Leave your complaints aside, yourself aside, and just describe it.
> Describe more about this gesture. What are you showing with your hands?

When the case does not naturally lead any further then ask the same question in a different way. Repeat the question until the words or expressions do not lead any further. Go back to the previous word or expressions with energy, or ask again: How does it affect you?

To move the patient from Level 2 (Fact) to Level 3 (Emotion), explore:

> Feelings denied;
> Past feelings;
> Opposite feelings;
> Avoided feelings;
> Go to level 4, Delusion then return to level 3, Emotion.

Once there is enough information with energy and details about the Chief Complaint or if there is no other information with energy to lead us further at the Fact level, then the homeopath needs to move ahead to the next possible level. If the case becomes completely stuck, then use a bypass, which will be explained later in the chapter.

Level of Emotion

At Level 3, Emotion, the homeopath explores the patient's feelings. The patient will talk about sadness, anger, irritation, fear, tension, worry, joy, happiness, and so forth, which are associated with the Chief Complaint or refer to a situation that is bothering them. Get the feelings qualified and elicit the peculiar feelings. Examine the situations in which these emotions arise. Look for language of delusion and sensation. What are the feelings? What is the quality of the feelings? What is peculiar? How does this affect you? See how the emotions are perceived and experienced.

If the patient doesn't give intense feelings, ask about some examples or some situation where these emotions were felt intensely. If the patient mentions some situation spontaneously, ask about the emotions experienced in that situation. Go further and see how the situation and emotions were perceived (Delusion level). If the patient mentions feelings that are too general and not specific enough, tell her to use more words and to be more concrete.

Usually the practitioner can apply an emotion that a person strongly and spontaneously denies. Ask the client to describe the feeling further even if she continues to deny it. For example, a person says, "Ghosts do not scare me." The question would be "Tell me about ghosts." Then the homeopath should continue to probe into the issue with ghosts keeping in mind that there might be a fear of ghosts, which the patient is denying. When a patient denies information, keep the denial in mind and see if it becomes relevant in another context in the case. For example, a patient says, "I am not a coward." The practitioner would probe and try to understand how cowardice is an issue for her in the rest of the case. Denial is often seen when feelings are compensated.

Some of the questions to ask at Level 3 to move the case along are:

> Describe your feelings.
> Use more words. The feeling is very general. Be more specific. Use other words.
> Give an example of a situation where you felt these emotions.
> What do you do in response to the emotions?

If the patient doesn't go any further, ask the same question in a different way. Go back to the previous word, which had energy or a strong gesture. Ask again, "Give one example or a situation where you had the same feeling." Explore exciting, denied or avoided situations in the patient's life. The practitioner can ask about an event that is about someone else that they are particularly sensitive to. Ask the patient to imagine a situation that would have that feeling, even if they haven't experienced it in their life. Books, movies, hobbies are also areas where emotions may surface. At the level of

Emotion, it is also possible to find out about situations they are worried about or might feel could happen. Similes and metaphors are also ideas worth looking into at this level.

At the level of Emotion it is not important to know why the patient is angry. The homeopath wants to understand the complete phenomena of his anger, which arises from delusion, sensation, and energy. This exploration of all the levels will reveal the complete truth.

To move the patient from level 3 (Emotion) to level 4 (Delusion), explore:

> Situations denied;
> Past exciting situations;
> Avoided situations;
> Projected situations;
> Anticipated situations;
> Sensitivity to others' situations;
> Interests like books, movies, etc.;
> Similes or metaphors.

When a person cannot get past the level of Emotion and the practitioner has explored all avenues of open-ended questioning, then consider using a bypass to go to a deeper level.

Level of Delusion

Delusion is the level where it is possible to see how the emotions are perceived and how the patient views her situations. Involuntary expressions and many dreams will take the patient to the level of Delusion. Look for the sensations, gestures, commonly used metaphors, visual images and imaginary scenarios. At this level the patient commonly uses the words "it is like…" or "as if…"

At this level it could have taken a lot of patience and faith before the patient will express a delusion. Sometimes the patient can get frustrated from being asked the same question repeatedly. Reassure the patient and keep asking the same question in different ways.

If the patient is not going deeper, then go back to the previous words that had energy. Explore intense or stressful situations in the patient's life, dreams, interests, hobbies, fears, fantasies, or any book, story, movies, television serials that come spontaneously to the client's mind.

Common questions to ask at the level of Delusion are:

> Please describe the situation.
> How did you perceive the situation?
> It was as if … (pause)?
> Describe more the experience.
> What does it feel like?

What picture comes to mind? If I ask you to draw a picture on a piece of paper, what would the image look like?
Give some examples.
Please describe an intense situation.
Describe what you are showing with your hands.
What would be an opposite situation or reaction?

At the level of Delusion there may be some commonly used metaphors, such as: I feel shattered; I felt stabbed in the back. Try to elicit precise images or imaginary situations. It is important to seek the unique perspective of the patient and not pay much attention to common clichés unless they are repeated over and over, have energy and relate to other aspects of the case. The homeopath can have the patient think about what would have happened in a past situation, or ask: "What is the worst thing that could have happened?" For example, what would have happened if your mother died? Sometimes a whole imaginary scene will be told when a patient describes what they are showing with their gestures. For example, a man pacing and stomping around the room will say, "I feel like a caged animal."

If the patient jumps back to the level of Fact or Emotion, then bring the client back to the point of delusion by asking, "How did you experience that situation?"

To move the patient from level 4 (Delusion) to level 5 (Sensation) explore:

The sensation in the Chief Complaint;
Hand gestures;
Physical or emotional sensations or consequences of an intense experience;
Similes or metaphors;
Opposite sensations (usually pleasant);
Opposite reactions to a situation.

When a person gets stuck at the level of Delusion and only gives images and pictures, but can not give the sensation, then the practitioner will have to use a bypass to get to the deeper levels.

Level of Sensation

Eventually the homeopath needs to bring the patient to the level of Sensation where non-human expressions are used. The patient will focus progressively on specific sensations, which will lead to a Vital Sensation at the level of Sensation. At this level, the homeopath will also be able to confirm the kingdom.

If the patient gives clear expressions of sensitivity and reaction, and on further probing explains the sensation very well with more images and examples, the patient could need a plant remedy. For example, if the patient says she feels tied and bound, then the homeopath could think of a plant remedy. If the patient expresses no specific sensations or a large variety of sensations, or no sensitivity at all, but personifies the disease by projecting issues of victim-aggressor, hierarchy or attractiveness, the case could belong to the animal kingdom. For example, if the patient says he feels cornered as if something is coming to shred him, then this could be animal kingdom. If the issues brought up by the patient are problems of structure (within themselves, in relationships, at work), or performance, then it could be a mineral case. For example, the patient, who needs a mineral remedy says her life is falling apart, she can't keep herself together, and she feels like she's floating through space.

One way of eliciting sensations is for the homeopath to ask how emotional phenomena are experienced physically. For example, a patient feels grief and the homeopath asks: How do you feel it physically? She replies it is a broken and splintering sensation. If it is an intense physical phenomenon, the homeopath needs to explore how it is felt mentally.

The common questions the practitioner can ask at the level of Sensation are:

Tell me more about the sensation or experience you described.
Describe more what you are showing with your hands.
How do the sensations or experience feel physically in that situation?
What did you feel in your head, chest and body,
    when you talked about this emotion?
Describe any similes or metaphors.
What were the sensations in a past circumstance?
What were the sensations in an intense situation or complaint?
Describe your experience more, not the complaints, just the sensation.
Are there any modalities in this sensation?
What is the opposite sensation?

When the homeopath asks more about the sensation and other information is spoken about, it is possible that this sensation will not lead to anything. However, when new images and words are related to the same essential theme, then this is a sign that the case is going in the right direction. Tracing the sensation further will lead to the kingdom (animal, plant, mineral or nosode), the sub-kingdom (plant family, animal group, and possibly mineral row and stage) and any source information or ideas that might indicate the specific substance required by the patient. The level of Sensation is where accurate language for the kingdom will be necessary to make a distinction. At the level of Delusion the patient may use kingdom language that does not represent the deepest state for them. Patients often express many kingdoms and it is important to take the patient to the level of Sensation for clarification of the kingdom.

Also at this level of Sensation, when the practitioner asks the patient how they experience the Vital Sensations, the language of the miasm will be expressed. Sometimes the patient will repeat the sensations of the Vital Sensation, however, with probing the miasmic language will be evident. For example, the homeopath asks: How do you experience these piercing, poking, sharp sensations? The patient replies that he tries to ignore it, avoid it, actually never talks about it. This answer would indicate the Sycotic miasm. It is the degree, depth and quality as well as how the patient copes with their Vital Sensations that reveal the miasm. The language of the patient's miasm occurs at all levels and can be further confirmed at the level of Sensation.

If the patient goes back to facts or emotions, bring her gently back to the point and ask about the sensation. If the patient goes back to the situation they already described, or to a new one, inquire how the situation was perceived and narrow her down to the sensation. If repeated attempts fail to give enough sensations then use a bypass.

To move the patient from level 5 (Sensation) to level 6 (Energy) explore:

> Movements and gestures of the patient;
> Sound, frequency and speed of speech;
> Repeated patterns or themes in the patient's interests or hobbies,
>   like music, art, dance, race cars;
> Similes or metaphors.

Use bypass when a person gets stuck at the level of Sensation in order to move to the deeper level of Energy.

Level of Energy

The Energy level is represented by gestures, direction, movement, pace, color and sound. Following the level of Sensation, the homeopath must keep focusing on the gestures, words or ideas associated with the Vital Sensation by investigating in detail until there is a complete sense of the Energy level. This is an exciting point in the case when the patient makes a leap into a universal consciousness that will seem surreal, totally imaginative, and descriptions may no longer be the same words for the Vital Sensation, but the source language for the substance or remedy required to deeply cure the patient. It is a significant stage in the casetaking but easily confused with the level of Delusion, especially in animal cases. So there must be caution in using this level to confirm a prescription.

If the patient returns to human-specific language, bring her back to the energy. The questions the homeopaths need to formulate at this level are to encourage the patient to describe more about the energy, the gesture, and the abstract language.

Observe the patient's movements (especially hand gestures), her speech (the sound, frequency, and speed) and anything else with energy. It is also important to notice if there are any repeated patterns in their interests (in music, art, dance, race cars, etc.). Detach the patient from human feelings or situations and take them to a non-human level of energy.

Many of the misconceptions about this method come from practitioners assuming they are at the level of Energy when in fact they are at the level of Delusion. A prescription using false "source" language or a situation described at the level of Delusion will often lead to a poorly prescribed remedy. For example, the patient says, "I feel like flying," and the homeopath assumes the patient needs a bird remedy. When the patient is at the level of Energy there is an experiential feeling in the consulting room, and the language is abstract and at the same time revealing a substance. Many times it is only after prescribing a successful remedy that it is clear what the source language is referring to in the case. It is not an easy level to understand or to make a guess at what the client is describing in order to make a prescription. It is a level that will make sense to the patient and brings deep awareness and may bring opportunities not yet explored thoroughly in homeopathy.

Exploring Dreams

The dreams of the patient always need to be explored in casetaking and are not always at the level of Delusion. What are the significant dreams now and in the past, especially during childhood? Are there any repetitive dreams? What is the main action in the dream? What is the sensation in the dream? Do not ignore or interpret dreams, but trace the feelings in the dreams and get the exact description of all the elements in the dreams.

If the dream is about a specific incident that really happened in life, find out what the impact of the real incident had on the patient. Was the patient's reaction appropriate to the situation or not? If the reaction to the situation was reasonable in real life then the dream is not important. If the reaction was disproportionate, then the feelings in the dream and in the situation should be noted.

If the client had a pleasant dream, try to find out how the patient would like things to be in her life. What is her perception of her present situation? Is her current experience similar or opposite to the dream? If the dream is unpleasant, then find out if the client has the same or opposite feeling in life.

If in the dream the patient sees someone or something else go through an intense experience, then the feelings brought up in the dream will be about the patient and useful to explore and understand. Often times in these projected dreams the intensity of sensations can be blunted.

In symbolic dreams it is possible to look for the rubric directly in the repertory. This symbol may be directly connected to the source of the remedy.

Bypass

Compensation of disease can fixate patients at specific levels, and bypasses enable the homeopath to lead the patient to deeper levels where they are no longer compensated (levels of Delusion, Sensation and Energy). If, after extensive open-ended questioning, the patient is stuck and is not able to reveal emotions, delusions, sensations or energy in the case, then a bypass will be necessary. When using a bypass, the homeopath is looking for anything unique or different, which could be a Vital Sensation and ties in with any sensations or themes uncovered from the Chief Complaint. Each area used as a bypass is examined in order to find the connections in the case.

Interests, fears, fascinations, childhood and exciting situations are the first themes to explore for a bypass. Dreams can also be used as a bypass when they do not flow naturally from the chief complaint. If these areas of eliciting unique perceptions in the patient do not work, then the homeopath needs to explore the patient's personality, aims, relationships, work, fantasies or religion. The homeopath asks a direct question in one of these areas in the hope that it will open the case into to the levels of Delusion, Sensation or Energy.

Bypasses are emergency techniques and should be avoided as long as the patient is flowing from level to level even if it is not in sequential order. If bypasses are misused, the homeopath can confuse the case and explore sensations that do not actually connect to the chief complaint. All the previous techniques of exploring the various levels, and how to move from level to level, are used depending of what is elicited from the patient when these subjects are explored. An effort is made once a Vital Sensation is recognized from a bypass to connect it to the chief complaint and any other problems in the patient's life.

A patient with extensive pathology may not express energy directly or have any meaningful gestures or characteristic expressions to work with. In that case, the bypasses may allow the homeopath to go deep into the case and come to the level of Sensation and Energy.

Interests

The homeopath may find the opposite sensation to the Vital Sensation when a patient pursues an interest or hobby actively. For example, a patient is into racing cars, the desire for speed might be the opposite sensation of stagnation, which is the Vital Sensation of the case. If it is a more passive interest then the same sensation may be found in the chief complaint. For example, a patient enjoys knitting which is the same as the restlessness in the Vital Sensation. An interest or hobby may be evoked by asking about books, movies or stories they love or hate.

The questions to ask about interests and hobbies are:

> What hobbies do you pursue with enthusiasm?
> What aspect of it appeals to you the most?
> What feeling do you get from the hobby?
> What does your hobby signify for you?
> What books, movies or stories do you enjoy or hate?
> Is there anything you deliberately avoid or hate?
> Try and elicit the feeling behind it.

Keep asking about the hobby until the same sensation as that in the Chief Complaint is found or the opposite becomes apparent.

Fears

The homeopath can ask about specific fears and probe a specific fear and how it is perceived. In the bypass it is necessary to understand how the fear is related to the sensation of the chief complaint. For example, the patient has a trembling sensation when she sees a snake and in the Chief Complaint there is the sensation of trembling when she has acid reflux. Now the sensation of trembling has to be explored to the level of Sensation to confirm it is a Vital Sensation and useful for prescribing a remedy.

The questions to ask about fears are:

> What fears do you have? If the patient denies a fear then examine that one too.
> Probe the fear and the feeling behind it.
> What kind of threat is it?
> Describe the situation when the fear is felt intensely.
> Where do you experience the fear?
> How do you experience the fear?
> With this fear what do you experience in your head, chest, body or mind?
> What is the emotional and physical sensation in that situation?
> What action do you take in response to the fear?
> Examine fears from childhood.

Fascinations

Examine the fascination or obsession in depth and find out the feelings behind it. Any extreme fascination will also have a strong fear or aversion. Try to see how the fascination relates to a sensation. How does the patient express the fascination in her life? For example, a patient has a fascination with aliens and also fears them.

Childhood

A crucial sensation and its expression, as well as its opposite, could be found in the patient's childhood. The questions that can be used are:

> What was your nature in childhood?
> What kind of relationships did you have in childhood?
> What were you sensitive to in childhood?
> How was a particular situation perceived in childhood?
> Were there any stressful or upsetting incidents in your childhood?

Exciting situations

Explore any stressful situation and see how it connects to a Vital Sensation or a sensation from the Chief Complaint. Try to see what happened from the perspective of the patient, how she felt, and avoid the story of what actually happened. Details unseemingly related to the story can be bypasses to other levels. For example, a patient relating an incident of being attacked mentions the weird shape of the mugger's hat. The best places to explore exciting situations are those that occurred at the time the pathology appeared, or difficult situations that ended when the pathology began.

The questions that can be asked are:

> Was there any major stress at the time the pathology appeared?
> Did any stress disappear when the pathology began?
> What usually creates stress for you?
> Do you avoid any situations?
> What situations or incidents have been the most stressful or upsetting in your life?
> What did you feel?
> How did you react?
> Is there any situation you remember from your childhood that upset you greatly?
> How did you perceive or experience the situation?

Patient's Personality

The homeopath can explore various aspects of the patient's personality and how it connects to a Vital Sensation. What is her typical behavior? Have the patient describe relatives and friends, which if it is intensely portrayed, then the unique descriptions can be applied to the patient.

Work

The patient's work and her perception of it can also connect to the Vital Sensation. Try to confirm the same sensation or its opposite with other parts of the case. The questions that can be asked are:

> Is there any stress at work?
> What aspects of the job do you find good?
> What are the problems at work?
> Why did you choose this work?

Relationships

The practitioner can also try to understand the patient's connections with her family, friends or important people in her life. What do the relationships mean to her? How do the relationships fulfill her? Find out what is peculiar in the relationship.

The questions that can be asked are:

> Who do you relate to and how?
> What do you like or dislike about this person?
> What is your attitude towards this person?
> Is there any stress in the relationship?
> If there is a stress, then do you want to continue this relationship?
>   Why or why not?
> If there is loss of a relationship, what does the loss mean to you?

Fantasies

See how their hopes and aspirations connect to the case, which will be the opposite of their delusion and fears. The questions the homeopath can ask are:

> What do you fantasize about?
> What are your hopes and aspirations?

Aims

It is a good approach to ask children what they want to be when they grow up. With adults this question can be a way to find out what they sincerely longed for which did not happen. The question to ask an adult would be:

> As a child what did you want to be when you grew up?

Religion

It is better to ask the patient what does religion or spiritual pursuits mean to her rather than finding out about her interests in this area of her life. The question to ask could be: What does religion, spirituality or philosophy mean to you?

All information understood from a bypass has to be reconfirmed in other aspects of the case, especially in regards to the Chief Complaint, dreams, other complaints or situations.

Conclusion

In this method of casetaking less time is spent at the level of Fact and Emotions and more attention is given to the level of Delusion, Sensations and Energy. Many prescriptions were based in the past on emotions and delusions, but now patients are given the possibility to articulate deeper sensations through casetaking, which when they receive a remedy prescribed at the level of Sensation and Energy act very deeply. Although the level of Energy is mostly un-chartered territory at this time, it is truly an amazing experience to explore it with the patient. The 7th Level is currently a concept only, however, patients do give energy from all levels all the time.

When the homeopath observes a patient closely in this method of casetaking, the patient will give the entire range of the seven levels throughout the case. The system of levels works as a progression or a dynamic evolution from undifferentiated to more differentiated sensations, which are recognized as Vital Sensations and represent the unique state of the patient. Pathology can have the effect of disrupting the patient's awareness of the different levels so that the connecting these levels together in the patient's consciousness already initiates the healing process.

E. LEVELS IN POTENCIES AND FOLLOW UPS

Potency

The potencies in this new method are determined by understanding the level in which the patient mostly experiences their Chief Complaint and daily life. For example, if the patient focuses on a diagnosis, then the homeopath would consider prescribing a 6c remedy. If the patient only wants to talk about the complaint itself then the potency would be 30c. If the patient is mainly expressing emotions concerning the problem, then it would be 200c. The patient lives at the level of Delusion then the potency would be 1M. There are cases where the patient primarily experiences their life at the level of Sensation so 10M would be given. Level of Energy would be a 50 M, and so forth.

Levels & Potency:

Level – 1   6c
Level – 2   30c
Level – 3   200c
Level – 4   1 M
Level – 5   10M
Level – 6   50M
Level – 7   CM

It is important to know if the person is feeling the sensation locally or generally, often the sensation is the same, but where the patient feels it will determine the potency. The patient may describe vividly all the levels, or focus on the level before or after the one she needs. The homeopath needs to understand the level that the patient experiences daily and prescribe at that level.

Follow-Ups

The potencies will also change as the patient moves to different levels during the treatment. In the follow up, the patient may need a lower potency because she went from the level of Delusion to Emotion. For example, after several months of treatment the patient has the same state but moves from the level of Delusion to the level of Emotion and needs the same remedy at a lower potency.

In the follow up listen to how the patient explains the current state of their Chief Complaint. For example:

Level 1: The patient will say her blood sugar has gone up (Name).

Level 2: The patient will say my pain is better locally (Fact).

Level 3: The patient will say I am better generally and feeling less irritable (Emotion).

Level 4: The patient will say I don't feel in a tunnel any more; I'm released (Delusion).

Level 5: The patient will say that I don't feel that heaviness any more, I'm much lighter (Sensation).

Level 6: The patient will say she feels energetic and can bounce up and down (Energy).

The homeopath needs to assess if the state is the same and at what level the patient is currently experiencing her Chief Complaint. One of the best areas to see if the state is the same and how deeply the remedy is acting is to take the patient back to the level of Sensation and find out how strongly the patient is experiencing that sensation or has it changed dramatically. It is possible to ask the patient directly how much change has been noticed in that sensation. This information will help to confirm the prescription or give indications that the remedy needs to be changed. The spontaneous way that the patient relates to her Chief Complaint can be assessed by the homeopath to determine the specific level at which the patient is currently living. In this follow up the homeopath can assess the situation and either wait, repeat the same potency or change it depending on how the patient relates to their problems.

F. COMMON PITFALLS

One of the most common pitfalls for homeopaths is to jump too quickly into the case by repeating back specific words or a word from the patient without seeing it confirmed repeatedly. The homeopath has to wait, listen and observe until the energy pattern is clearly seen and some indications of a Vital Sensation are recognized before repeating a particular phrase or words back to the patient. For example: A young girl has problems with her best friend and she says that she has to chase after her friend who runs away all the time. Chase and running are expressions that hold energy in the case and could give indications of the kingdom, however, be careful not to pull them out until there are more and more expressions that confirm the sensation.

Another pitfall is to ask about a specific word. In the beginning of the case it is better to repeat back a number of words that the patient has spoken so that the patient can choose what is more significant.

It is often confusing to know if the sensation is local at the Fact level or at the level of Sensation. For example: the patient says he has a stinging pain in the left eye (local and at the Fact level) and then the homeopath uses this expression as a Vital Sensation or even possibly a sensation for selecting the remedy, which may be inaccurate.

The levels should be found directly and not by using bypasses unless absolutely necessary. Keep the questions open-ended and follow the suggestions of the types of questioning. In more compensated patients, bypasses may be needed and then consider prescribing for one level lower than how they express it. For example a patient who seems to live their life at the level of Emotion may need a 30c (Fact level) if the homeopath requires a number of bypasses to get the case.

There is an inherent difficulty in this method of confusing the level of Delusion with the level of Energy. Many excellent prescriptions will not require taking the patient to the level of Energy, or if the patient does go to the level of Energy the homeopath many not understand the patient's source language. The level of Sensation is an excellent confirmation of the kingdom, sub-kingdom and possibly the choice of the remedy. Whenever possible use the repertory and Materia Medica to confirm prescriptions, seek possibilities or rule out a remedy choice.

The common pitfalls are:

> Jumping too quickly into the case;
> Choosing one word to explore;
> Confusing a sensation that is local (Fact level) and general (Sensation level);
> Using a bypass when not needed;
> Confusing level of Delusion and level of Energy;
> Not researching known remedies to either confirm or rule out a
>   prescription.

G. SAMPLE CASES
By Melissa Burch, CCH

CASE 1

CASE 1 TEXT of CASE Woman in her 70's.	CASE ANALYSIS
Client: Well, amazingly so. It was interesting to do the review that you suggested on your website. And in doing that, I realized I have come a long way in the last two years.	
Homeopath: So, what would you like to change? I mean, if homeopathy could do anything for you, what would you like to see changed?	*Identifying the Chief Complaint.*
Well, you had talked about living at a whole new level, and really, that's what I'm after.	*Chief Complaint – I want to Live at a Whole New Level.*
Okay, so what would that mean for you?	*When clients do not have Specific Problems and instead come in for General Wellness – ask them to define what this means for them? What would be the Experience of "Living at a Whole New Level?"*
A lot more of a higher sense of awareness. A lot more of being able to live from a center of love all of the time without <u>getting sucked into the nuances of everyday life</u>.	
Okay, so talk a little bit more about this living life without getting sucked into the nuances.	*Stay General until you Understand what the Chief Complaint is.*
It was interesting for me to drive the Mass Pike, and then Route 2, and then Massachusetts Avenue. I haven't been to Cambridge in many years, but I lived here for a year. And to have somebody honk-honk-honk at me because my car cut off at a stop	

CASE 1 TEXT of CASE Woman in her 70's.	CASE ANALYSIS
light. And I started to get sort-of tense (*HG/BG*) of two fists. I realized that I was starting to get <u>sucked</u> into that person's energy or my old energy that says, "I have to do things all right." (*HG*) But then I could consciously come back into my heart center and say, "that person may be having a hard day too. I don't have to be there right at 5 minutes to one. Let's relax here." And I've gotten in the habit of <u>sending out love to each one of my cells</u> when I find myself like this, but I don't always remember. And suddenly I'll find myself all caught up in emotion. For example, I was tired the other evening when I was with my grandchildren. My granddaughter was getting very silly—she's six. And I started to speak very sharply, but then I thought, "that's my problem, not hers. I don't need to <u>pour out that energy onto her</u>." (*HG – one hand sweeps*) So, again, <u>I had to send love to all of my nerves and cells and everything</u> (*HG circles by head*). But it is very difficult to stay there—in the midst of interactions with people in everyday life. When it's just me, I'm fine. But usually it's in the interactions with other people.	
So a little bit more about sending love into the nerves and cells. What is that like for you? How do you experience that?	
Well, it started with a dream I had. I've always been devoted to Jesus, because my father was a minister. And in the dream, Jesus was there and I was having a conversation with him. He said, "if you want to teach your grandchildren to meditate, here's what you can do: You can sit with them and say to them, 'imagine Jesus,' who my granddaughter is just absolutely devoted to, 'imagine that Jesus is right in front of you and just <u>sending out waves and waves and waves of love</u> (*HG/BG*) from his heart to your heart. And then take that love and	

CASE 1 TEXT of CASE Woman in her 70's.	CASE ANALYSIS
distribute it all over the body'." So I decided I would try it myself. And it's been my meditation every morning since then, and this was a couple of years ago. I have my meditation every morning when I wake up. It's wonderful. And so this consciously sending out love that *is* me, but beyond me, too. I'm a conduit for it, but I'm it too. And I sat down with my grandchildren and did that and they loved it! My grandson, who's turning 9, said, "Grandma, I can feel my heart and hear it and feel it getting warm, beating like that." It was wonderful. And my granddaughter just did it, and she thought it was great because Jesus was inside her, like this part of God was inside her. So that's where I got that idea.	
Okay, very good. The way we'll work together, I am going to keep asking you the same questions about this because you'll give me a new. . .	*Explaining the Process to the Client to Encourage them to go Deeper.*
Yes, that's what you did with the writing exercise.	
Right, right. Exactly. So, just a little bit more about this feeling of bringing in all the love and sending out waves into the heart.	*This "Sends Out Waves....." is a probable <u>Vital Expression</u>. She has used this Language in both her Daily Life (with the driving incident and her Granddaughter) and in the Spontaneously related Dream. Additionally there is Energy in the form of Gestures when she talked about this "Sending Out Love."* *<u>The Vital Expression is shaping up to include</u> "this send out to the cells," "send out in waves," "pour out," and "sucked in."*
Okay, well I know that I do, but I would like to be able to do it all the time, for all the people that I meet or who I'm with. Or let this be who I am, rather than just doing it	

CASE 1 TEXT of CASE Woman in her 70's.	CASE ANALYSIS
when I think about it. In other words, to do it all the time without thinking about it would be what I would like to be able to do.	
And do you have a Sensation with this? **Can you describe a Sensation when you do this?**	*Using this "Send Out the Waves, etc... as a Vital Expression, we now want to find out her Experience of this "Send Out Waves...." to Confirm Kingdom.* *When the Client is Intellectualizing or Caught Up in Ideas and Story — you can urge them to connect the Idea to a Sensation in the Body.* *"What is the Experience in the Body of this Idea you are describing to me?"*
Very similar to what my grandson described, I feel my heart (and I'd rather have it in my heart than in my head). I realized I am an emotion-based person. Anyway, I think it's the heart of the universe. It's sort of a warm feeling, a pulsing feeling, and, as I said before, it *is* me, but it is something bigger than me as well.	
Great, so it's a warm, pulsing feeling. Just use more words for that.	*Repeat Back the Client's Words in the Same Tone and Cadence they used and urge them to tell more.*
Okay, when I send it out, it's like a beacon sending out light in all directions (HG), only on these sort-of pulsing waves that go out in all directions. I've never really thought about this before. I just did it.	*The client confirms the Vital Expression of "Sending Out" by using it a third time.* *She gives us a Delusion first with "bigger than me" now with "like a beacon."* *"Pulsing Out in All Directions" is the Non Human Specific Language.*
Okay, a little bit more. It's like a beacon of light, but it's pulsing…	
Or like radio towers sending out sound waves that people who are tuned into the frequency	*Delusional Language-- we can see how the Delusions keep changing as she tries to describe*

CASE 1 TEXT of CASE Woman in her 70's.	CASE ANALYSIS
know exactly what it is. People who may not be on that <u>frequency</u> may sense that it's just something else, or they are just not aware of it. But, I do feel like it affects people even if they are not aware of it. Not that I'm trying to make people change, it's just that, to me, love is the ultimate emotion, and I am an emotion-based person, so…it's the greatest thing that I can experience. And so <u>to send that out</u> to other people is to be the ultimate experience.	*her Sensation.* *It is common that when you are on Delusional Level that the Delusional Images keep Changing.* *What is Common to her Delusions is that all these are Examples of things that "Send Out/Go Out/Pour Out" which definitely confirms this as the <u>Vital Expression</u>.*
I'm just going to keep asking you…you've been very descriptive, it's been very helpful. So it's like a frequency that some people are not aware of, but other people are affected by it. Just a little bit more about what you mean by that. It's like a radio tower sending out waves…	*Repeating Back her Vital Expression Language to find the Kingdom.*
I guess another analogy would be <u>waves on the ocean</u>. From throwing something in the water and it <u>sends out ripples</u>, (*HG of waves*) circular <u>ripples all the way out</u>. I think some are on the surface and people see them. Some are under the surface and they may not be seen, but I suppose that people who are in the water can feel them and they can be aware of it or not aware of it.	*Delusional Language but the Same Hand Gesture with All these Images of "Send Out," "Frequencies," "Waves," "Ripples."* *The Repeated Hand Gesture tells us we are in the Right Place.* *Now we need to Understand the Kingdom.*
And in the imagination, let's say, because you are so clear. How is this experience then, not so much in your situation, although you've described it beautifully, but this sort-of wave in the ocean or waves, frequencies coming through towers? How do you think that's experienced? A little bit more.	*Dissociate her from her Story and Situation and Focus on the Vital Expression and Non Human Specific Language to coax more Kingdom Language out of her.* *Kingdom Language So Far – Warm, Pulsating. Tuned In, Frequency.*
By me or by other people?	

CASE 1 TEXT of CASE Woman in her 70's.	CASE ANALYSIS
Just, even abstractly. It can be completely imaginative now.	
I guess, let's see. I think of the universe as being <u>full of this energy</u>. And I think of the universe as being full of this love energy. We just might not call it that. We call it <u>quantum</u> or we call it <u>protons</u>, (*HG*) or whatever we call it. And when something, in mechanistic terms, <u>excites that</u>, or (*HG -- waves*) <u>focuses that in one direction</u>, then it can affect <u>everything around it</u>. Because then if <u>it's a unified field, like air</u>, then something that is going through it will affect everything that it goes through. I guess that's the way I can describe it.	*Kingdom Language – All <u>this Language is</u> <u>Pointing to Something that is Not Really</u> "Matter" but Something that has an Effect on "Matter."* *This is <u>Imponderable</u>.* *The Remedy is Something that is <u>Energy in the Universe</u>.* *This is <u>SOURCE LANGUAGE</u>.*
Good. You're doing great. You're very clear.	
Well, this is very interesting to have to put words to it, pictures to it. I hadn't really thought about it.	
Yes, you're very clear.	
I have done it so much as a feeling, and not so much as an imagination, in the visual terms, and it's fascinating.	
And so if it's these quantum protons and it's got this mechanism, that gets excited, and then if gets focused on, and then it's like a field. So then these waves come through, just a little bit more.	*Repeat Back this Kingdom Language to urge her to go further.*
Okay, well something I've been pondering recently is the <u>manifestation</u>, a <u>physical manifestation</u> from imagination. Because my best friend and I, Cindy, are planning on starting a retreat center. And that's a big manifestation. And I've been thinking about	*Going Back to her Story but there is a Spontaneous Connection happening here – Pay Attention.*

CASE 1 **TEXT of CASE** **Woman in her 70's.**	CASE ANALYSIS
what is the <u>process of manifestation</u>. And it seems to me that this comes into play as if the love <u>energy goes out</u> into the sea (*HG of waves*), the ocean, whatever it is of love. And then with the image or the focus on the cottages we want, the community buildings we want, <u>sending that out</u> (*HG of waves*) every time it touches something that jives with that image, that it…<u>I'm not sure what the mechanism is</u>, but I connect with that. Or <u>whoever is sending out the energy</u>, the love, connects with that and then somehow I end up being connected like I am with you here. I mean this is an amazing synchronicity, to me. Who would have thought that going to East Brookfield would have brought me to Cambridge?	*Mechanism??*
So in your imagination, what is this mechanism then that you see?	
<u>Maybe like a magnet</u>, like ones that fit together, or are <u>drawn together</u>. (*HG – hand go together*) If they're focused on…you know, if I'm focused on an image, and then something that fits that image gets <u>drawn to me</u> or I to it. This is all very interesting. I've never really thought about it mechanistically before.	*Named a Possible Remedy – BUT, now you must listen for <u>WHAT DOESN'T FIT. IF EVERYTHING FITS – FINE OR SOMETHING ELSE COULD COME OUT</u>.*
You're doing very well. You're very clear. Now what happens then that sometimes you are reminded to do this, in situations where… like with the honking, what is that?	*Going back to the Chief Complaint – "Forgetting to Send Out the Love when Someone Honks "– a bit More of a Concrete Take on the Complaint than just wanting to Live at a Whole New Level.* *We need to see her put all the Pieces Together – <u>come back to Magnet</u> and then we can be Sure OR she could takes us Somewhere Else <u>and then we need to Reassess</u>.*
What is it that reminds me?	

CASE 1 TEXT of CASE Woman in her 70's.	CASE ANALYSIS
Well, or the experience when they were honking and you felt like…	
In the beginning, I would go home and sort-of review my day, and go, "oh, I didn't have to get all bent out of shape over that." Now looking at it, I realize that just by doing it over the last couple of years, I have become more aware of being able to do it *in* the situation instead of afterwards.	
So describe that. You used the words, "sucked in."	*From the first part of the Interview – another part of the Vital Expression. If we pick this – will she come back to the Same Place or take us Somewhere New.*
Yes, I did. I used the words sucked in.	
So what is that for you?	
Probably the <u>same kind of mechanism that I use when I send out love</u>, or love combined with images. I have a hunch that somebody else might be <u>sending out</u> an anger <u>wave</u>. And because I was exposed to that as I young child, I <u>tuned into</u> that. I was <u>drawn like a magnet to that</u> and went right back to my childhood and experienced the same fear or anger or whatever I had experienced before. So it was something I already knew and I think it's because that was <u>attracted to the other</u>. Because there have been times when someone was angry about something and I'm just sort-of scratching my head saying, "okay, alright, but I don't quite understand why they're angry about this." But if it touches some image in me, I guess, then <u>I get attracted to it</u> (*HG from earlier of hands going together*) and that image becomes what I'm experiencing in that moment.	*All the Same Language and Hand Gesture coming back – Tuned In, Mechanism, Send Out, Wave, Drawn In, Magnet. <u>Attracted</u> is New Word that comes in now.* *Now we just tune in and listen for Source Language Quality Words even though she may be talking at Story or Emotion Level – We Tune in Our Listening for <u>Source Quality Words</u> and Pursue these.*
Very good. Very, very clear. So just	*Repeat Back and Add in the New Word.*

CASE 1 TEXT of CASE Woman in her 70's.	CASE ANALYSIS
describe this a little bit more – (indicate the Gesture of Hands Going Together.) It's like a magnet, it's attracted, just a little bit more about what that is.	
For me, it's carried on feelings. When I was a child, my mother used to call me Moonie Mouse. I was very little, very tiny, and I had a lot of fear. I was afraid of this, I was afraid of that. She also called me Moonie Mouse, because I was always off in my imagination somewhere. So that was that part. But that mouse part, I had a lot of fears. I was afraid of other people. I was afraid of not doing the right thing. I was afraid of this, that, and the other. And anger in particular, I also had a lot of anger. I had a very bad temper. My father had several talks with me about that. He then he said he had it too, so. And again, I don't whether as an infant I <u>osmosed</u> his anger, or whether I had it already in my own nervous system. He has always says that my nervous system seems very much like his side of the family. Or whether it was just my experience. I don't know. Being very tiny and not able to control much in my life, I would get very fearful and very angry. And even up until the last few years, if I was not right on time for something that I was important to me, I would get really, really upset with myself. Angry at myself. Fearful that…I don't know, I don't know what I was fearful of. But that was why today was so lovely. I thought, well, she's not going to be angry with me if I'm ten minutes late. Why don't I just enjoy this? But I do sort-of feel that when somebody else is angry I go into the child mode of being fearful of not doing the right thing. I guess they become my father in me (*HG – hands drawn together*) and I become this little girl again and…	*Dropping Back into Story and Emotion but we are Listening for <u>Source Quality Words</u>.*

CASE 1 TEXT of CASE Woman in her 70's.	CASE ANALYSIS
What is this (*HG*)?	
This is the <u>attraction</u>. This is the anger, this is the person, this is me. And here is the person who is angry, and here is the person, me, who feels…I'm fearful and angry at myself because I haven't done the right thing. Either that I've done the wrong thing or that I haven't done the right thing. And so then this anger is <u>sending out all these waves</u> (*HG of waves*) of anger, and I'm <u>tuning into them</u> and <u>attracted</u> to it because that's what my past pattern was. And so if I can detach from this pattern and not be <u>magnetically drawn</u> to experiencing that situation emotionally. If I can step outside of it, well, then I can see that here's me and here's this man who's mad. Isn't that interesting. I think, "<u>send</u> love to both of them."	*Source Words* *Previous Language Coming Back in that Confirms All the Pieces coming Together.*
Right, because it is the same mechanism.	
Anyway, that's very interesting to think about.	
Very good. Very good. Okay. Let's talk about, not so much about you again, but just this mechanism, this attraction. Just describe it a little bit more. Not so much about your situation, but just what is this in general.	*Dissociate her Further – Get her Away from Story and Emotion and gather <u>More Source, Quality Words</u> to Confirm or Lead us Some Place Else*
I guess as human beings in physical bodies. At least for me, lots of things are carried on the emotions. And the nervous system reacts to emotions. It seems to me that patterns from childhood, or past lives if you believe in past lives, are triggered by things that happen in this life, especially when they happen early in life. And when you experience it one time, <u>you sort-of build a little circle of tape</u>. And then you experience it again, and that <u>tape comes back into play</u>. (*HG of this tape wrapping around*) But then <u>it builds another layer of</u>	*More Source Language Layered in the Story.*

CASE 1 **TEXT of CASE** **Woman in her 70's.**	CASE ANALYSIS
magnetic tape around it, and you experience it again and it builds a bigger…so you end up with this great big ball of magnetic memory tape. And then somebody else has their big ball of memory tape and begins to have similarities to your memory tape or the same emotions, or the same pattern, I guess I should say. Because this is anger, this is fear. That's not exactly the same, but based on this person's experience of having someone angry at them or exploding and angry and having someone fearful of them. And this person is having fear of this anger and then actually turns around and is angry with somebody else. This great big ball of memory tape gets bigger and bigger and bigger as those emotions are experienced again and again and again and again. Or I guess I could say the patterns get more deeply entrenched the more you experience it again and again and again. So you have to unwind your ball, I guess.	
And what is unwinding your ball then?	
Or else you have to step outside the ball and not be inside the ball while you're experiencing. I think that would be easier than trying to go back to each one of those memory tapes and to say, "okay, what was this," and to look at it from the outside, "what did it do?" I think that's what therapy probably does. Now that I think about it, I'd rather just step outside the whole ball and say, "sorry, there you go." Throw it into the river and let it dissolve.	
So if we were just going to abstract this for a little bit, there's this magnetic mechanism and then there's this magnetic ball.	*Dissociate – get her Away from Story and Repeat Back Words and Gestures.*
Yes, and the bigger it gets, the more it's drawn to another magnet that is that big too. It	

CASE 1 TEXT of CASE Woman in her 70's.	CASE ANALYSIS
becomes more and more of a <u>really heavy magnet</u> because it's got <u>more stuff there to draw</u>. The <u>bigger the magnet, the bigger the draw</u>. You know, the earth draws a lot more than a <u>tiny little magnet</u>. So the <u>more layers of magnetic memories that you're putting on it, the greater it attracts</u>.	*Everything Staying Consistent – Good Confirmation of the Remedy so Far.*
Okay, so just talk about magnets. Just what do you know about magnets?	*Now we have her tell us Everything about Magnets and Listen for WHAT DOESN'T FIT.*
About magnets?	*IF it ALL FITS – WE are on SOLID GROUND.*
Yes, everything you know about magnets.	
They <u>attract</u>. They <u>especially attract when they are with other magnets</u>, because each one has such a <u>strong pull</u>. That's interesting. That they <u>attract anything with iron in them, but iron is passive and is attractive</u>. <u>Magnets are active and attract</u> as well as being <u>attracted to other magnets</u>. That's an interesting concept. I haven't really thought about that. <u>So if you're just iron, you don't do any attracting, you're just attracted to</u>. <u>If you're a magnet, you attract, as well as being attracted to</u>.	*We ALSO Need to See All the Clues/Language come Back from Earlier in the Case as part of the Confirmation in Regards to Magnet.*
You're more the magnet.	*Must Also be Very Cautious when it seems Too Easy – Check, Double Check, Triple Check.*
I hadn't thought about that. Wow. Although I am very much <u>attracted</u> to spiritual things, growth and personal growth, positive emotions, and helpfulness to other people. And wherever I find those, I am <u>attracted</u> to them. So, in that sense I guess I would be the <u>iron</u> there.	*Goes Back to her Life but the Source Language Shines Through.*

CASE 1 TEXT of CASE Woman in her 70's.	CASE ANALYSIS
The iron becomes a magnet sometimes.	
Exactly. The interesting thing is that you have to <u>magnetize it by having it be around a magnet</u>. Now isn't that very interesting? I think that what I have found is that by meditating everyday and putting myself in that <u>love energy</u>, then I become more of that. So, yes, <u>I become more of a magnet, the more I am in that magnetic energy</u>. That's fascinating. Wow.	*Love Energy – Issue from the Chief Complaint comes Back in – Great Confirmation that it is All Coming Together.*
Great. Alright.	
Oh, and <u>if you want to be a really strong magnet, you become an electric magnet</u>. And to do that…my grandson and I were doing and experiment the other night. <u>You have to take iron and wrap</u>—again, you're wrapping, but it's got to be good stuff. <u>You're wrapping it with wire</u>. And there may be—what was Dan saying the other night at our alternative energy meeting? <u>1500 turns</u>. He was going to have to make <u>1500 turns with the wire around the magnet in order to make a really, really strong electro-magnet</u>. But then you not only have the <u>pull of a magnet</u>, but you also have, <u>if you turn on a current, it multiplies the draw. Many, many times. Just because you've wrapped these wires around it. So that there are magnetic balls</u> or <u>magnetic wraps that can affect you negatively</u>, but there are <u>also magnetic wraps that can affect you positively</u>. Hmmm. Very interesting.	*Here the Wrapping comes Back – PERFECT!!* *Strange Synchronicity with Grandson and Magnet – We are Right There.* *No Indication of One Pole or the Other – Must be the Whole Magnet.*
Very good. Very Interesting. Alright. Anything else about magnets?	
Not that I can think of right off the bat. Except that I would like to <u>power our retreat center with electromagnetic energy as much from the earth or from the love sea as I can</u>.	*Amazing……….*

CASE 1 TEXT of CASE Woman in her 70's.	CASE ANALYSIS
	Love of CC comes Back in Again.
	Remedy: magnetis poli ambo Potency: 1M

Overview: Client looking to shift consciousness, no physical complaint. Start by asking what shifting consciousness means for her. She names the substance (magnet), so have to be careful to listen for what doesn't fit – stay at level of potentiality. Case goes too fast, so go back to a concrete part of chief complaint to confirm, also explore another possible VE. Clients who live at energy/sensation level will often have direct experience with substance.

Chief Complaint: client wants to "live at whole new level"

Vital Expression: Sending out love, pour out, HG waves. "Sucked in" could have also been picked and is later explored to confirm.

Some question homeopath asks once VE is identified:

So, just a little bit more about this feeling of bringing in all the love and sending out waves into the heart.
Great, so it's a warm, pulsing feeling. Just use more words for that.
Can you describe a sensation when you do this?
And in the imagination, let's say, because you are so clear. How is this experience then, not so much in your situation, although you've described it beautifully, but this sort-of wave in the ocean or waves, frequencies coming through towers? How do you think that's experienced? A little bit more.
And so if it's these quantum protons and it's got this mechanism, that gets excited, and then it gets focused on, and then it's like a field. So then these waves come through, just a little bit more.
Let's talk about, not so much about you again, but just this mechanism, this attraction. Just describe it a little bit more. Not so much about your situation, but just what is this in general.

Kingdom Language: Imponderable (*something that has an affect on matter but isn't really matter*)

It's sort of a warm feeling, a pulsing feeling, and, as I said before, it *is* me, but it is something bigger than me as well.
Or like radio towers sending out sound waves that people who are tuned into the frequency know exactly what it is.

I think of the universe as being full of this energy. And I think of the universe as being full of this love energy. We just might not call it that. We call it quantum or we call it protons, or whatever we call it. And when something, in mechanistic terms, excites that, or (*HG -- waves*) focuses that in one direction, then it can affect everything around it. It's energy. I see the universe as full of energy. Although, I tend to see the universe as full of love energy, but how does it get misdone into anger energy?

Source Language:

Because then if it's a unified field, like air, then something that is going through it will affect everything that it goes through.
I become more of a magnet, the more I am in that magnetic energy. That's fascinating. But then you not only have the pull of a magnet, but you also have, if you turn on a current, it multiplies the draw. Many, many times. Just because you've wrapped these wires around it. So that there are magnetic balls or magnetic wraps that can affect you negatively, but there are also magnetic wraps that can affect you positively.
I would like to power our retreat center with electromagnetic energy as much from the earth or from the love sea as I can.
The anger, it's like a swirling ball of energy, only it's very loosely attached.
When I talked about magnetic memories winding around each other so that you have this great big ball, something triggers it to spin around and trigger all the memories it wants.

Energy Language:

Maybe like a magnet, like ones that fit together, or are drawn together. (*HG – hand go together*) If they're focused on...you know, if I'm focused on an image, and then something that fits that image gets drawn to me or I to it.

Remedy: magnetis poli ambo (magnet)

Dose: 1M

Case Management and Outcome: In first week after casetaking, client went through every major disease symptom from her life BEFORE even taking the remedy. In second week (no remedy) she relived her emotional experiences. On remedy, she has become a powerful manifester.

CASE 2

CASE 2 of WOMAN with MS TEXT of CASE	ANALYSIS of CASE
Homeopath: What is the main problem for you now? What is affecting you the most?	
Client: I have multiple sclerosis (MS). If I could reduce the fatigue—which is severe—increase my energy, and get rid of the muscle pain I've had in my right leg, (I've had it for two years, it's an overuse injury). I would be very happy.	*Listening for Chief Complaint*
Okay, so tell me as much as you can about this fatigue and pain in right leg and its overuse.	*Chief Complaint*
Well, fatigue is a symptom of MS anyway. But mine is severe. I don't know if it's due to medications, I'm on a number of medications. I'm off the medications that may have been contributing to it. I don't know what it is – some imbalance in my system. Always had fatigue but this is severer. May be tied into dragging this leg around..... (Tea Arrives)........ My left side is the side that's affected by my MS. And it is an overuse injury in my right leg after 30 years of carrying the weight for the other leg. And they haven't been able to diagnose it until recently. I was going to a physical medicine doctor for a year and a half, and then I went to a physical medicine doctor at the MS clinic who thought that it has to do with my toes compensating for a weak ankle or the weakness. So they have me in what they call a foot-op brace on the right leg, which is a little insert under the laces of my shoes that attaches to a band around my ankle. And it pulls my leg up, my foot-op, so I don't have to do anything. And that actually has given me much more relief walking. I'm more comfortable walking. I'm not comfortable sitting, and especially lying, because I can't get my foot in a neutral position. I have a resting splint, that looks like I came from some planet, but I have to ice it a lot. And I was on different medications before that made me sick, but didn't do a thing	*Mostly Fact Level with Some Local Sensation (dragging) and Delusion (some imbalance in my system). Too early to focus on these words or you risk narrowing the case and going down a long and misleading path.*

CASE 2 of WOMAN with MS TEXT of CASE	ANALYSIS of CASE
for the pain, so I'm off of them now. I, also, which I didn't mention, have a totally arthritic left shoulder.	
So, just to talk again, more about this fatigue in the striding leg, this brace that you have, and then at night you have a resting split, just more. I'm going to keep asking you the same questions because I'm trying to understand how you experience this fatigue and this overuse.	*Urge the client to give more details about the Fatigue and Leg Pain (CC).* *Brief explanation of the Process.*
Sure, well, I have insomnia, so I take Ambien, because they finally decided that it was more important with MS that I get the sleep that I need. So I take Ambien. And it does make me feel good, but within a couple of hours, I'm tired again. And I can maybe do something for two or three hours, and then I need to rest. And it's <u>extremely frustrating, very frustrating</u>.	*Fact Level* *Emotional Level*
And how do you experience this tiredness? What is the sensation in your body of this tiredness?	*Focus on the Experience in the Body of the Chief Complaint.*
It's, I need to stop and just relax, put my feet up. Sometimes I can work through it, sometimes I just <u>force</u> myself to do what I'm doing. <u>It's annoying. It just really interferes with what I want to do.</u>	*How the Chief Complaint Affects her Life.*
And the sensations in the body? Annoying, and this tiredness, and when you have to force yourself?	*Urging her to get into the body and tap into the Sensation of the Chief Complaint.*
Do I feel sensations in the body? No, I don't think so. I'm not aware. No, I think it's just more, I'm frustrated.	*She denies Sensation and returns to Emotion.*
Okay, and how do you experience frustrated?	
Probably getting a little bit down, getting a little depressed. I seem to spend more time lying down, trying to take care of the fatigue, than doing what I really want to do.	*Emotion Level*

CASE 2 of WOMAN with MS TEXT of CASE	ANALYSIS of CASE
So you may not have consciously experienced the sensations in the body, but I'm going to take you so that you can start to put words to it. Because that's part of it. I mean, homeopathy has many levels of prescriptions, so one is a diagnostic, you know. We could find the best remedy for MS, but it won't work. Homeopathy is terrible at that. We might get it, but. . .it would be a shot in the dark, most likely. And then there's another level of understanding what is particular in these MS symptoms, and that is one very important piece of information. And then there are other levels, like the emotional. You brought in the feelings of frustration and even feeling a little down about it. And then there are even more levels. And one of the levels that really helps to get a deep remedy is to start to become aware of your sensations in the body.	*Client is stuck on the Fact Level. The homeopath has asked repeatedly to talk about her sensation and experience of the Chief Complaint and she continues to give fact and even denies Sensation.* *So, by explaining the process to the client, you are in essence contracting with her. You are explaining the goal of the casetaking process and getting her consent to go to a Deeper Level...*
Okay.	
And you may not be aware of it now, in daily life, but you actually are aware of them in a way. So that's what I'm going to try to understand a little more. You've mentioned a lot of things with this tiredness, the feeling a little down, the frustration, the overuse of the right leg.	*Refocus the client on the Chief Complaint.*
Yes, there is also a fear of, "oh, what if I'm out driving and I get tired and I can't do this?"	*She gives a situation where the Chief Compliant affects her life.*
Okay, so let's take that example. So you're out driving and you get tired, and then you have this fear. What's the experience of that like for you?	*Go with the situation and ask for the Experience in this example she has given.*
It's, "What do I do? Oh no, what do I do? <u>Here it comes again</u>." And really, what I can do is pull over and rest. Usually I just turn on the air conditioner. And <u>I just really try to focus</u> when I'm like that and I have to be somewhere. And I don't know if <u>I fall back on it also</u>. (*HG one hand shows fall back*) <u>Sometimes I wonder if I'm</u>	*Spontaneously gives Gesture and an Expression -- "fall back." This "fall back" is the experience of her Chief Complaint. This appears to a <u>Vital Expression</u> since it is the first sign of Energy and Gesture and Non Human Specific Language.*

CASE 2 of WOMAN with MS TEXT of CASE	ANALYSIS of CASE
actually falling back on that.	*Let's see if it takes us deeper........*
So you can focus and then you can fall back on this. Just talk about this focus and falling back.	
Yes. If I have to go somewhere, if I have to do something, I just talk myself into the fact that, "I have to do this." You know, I can rest later, I can rest before, but I have to do this (*HG Same as Above*). And I can usually do what I have to do.	*Repeated Gesture of the 'fall back" hints that there is enough energy here to pursue this as a Vital Expression.*
Talk about just this (HG), you're doing this gesture. What is this?	*Focus on the Gesture – the only Sign of Energy in the Case thus far – if it is a Vital Expression, it should move the case deeper...*
I guess it's trying to will my body to do what I want it to do. And you can't do that with MS. But that's the kind of control that I'd like to have over it. And I don't have. It's so unpredictable. And I can't tell when I'm going to be tired.	*Earlier she mentions force her body to do things....*
I'm going to keep asking the same questions. So it's this (HG). And the focus. And you can, if you have to, will your body to do it. So just use more words to describe that.	
I guess I just won't accept anything but what I need to do. Maybe it's putting too high of standards on it, that I have to do this. I guess there's the fear of giving into it. I think this is why I say, "Focus—you can't give into this." Because it happens all the time. And I'm afraid I'll never, ever get out. And I mean, I'm always up, I always get dressed. I've never been one to stay in bed. But I may stay on the couch, you know. I may not make it very far. And it's just really debilitating, because it prevents me from wanting to make plans. Or at least when I make plans, making sure people know there is a possibility I will cancel. And I don't. I try not to do that because I just don't want that. You know, I have a lot of really good friends and I don't want to have a reputation of, "don't make	*Story and Emotion.......*

CASE 2 of WOMAN with MS TEXT of CASE	ANALYSIS of CASE
plans because Nancy will cancel." Even though everybody knows that I can't control that.	
So a little bit more about this focus, willing your body.	
I think it's just my way of trying to have control over my body. It's my way of having control, saying, "Okay, Nancy, if you concentrate on what you have to do, maybe the fatigue won't interfere." You know, "you have to do this."	
And the sensation in the body of this? This having to do it, the focus, willing the body to do it. Maybe you just have to close your eyes, even, and try to imagine.	*Again – trying to get her into her body and out of the Story and away from the Emotions.*
Yes, I am doing that. Maybe more tired.	
More tired. So how do you experience more tired?	
Oh, just everything is an effort. Everything is an effort. Everything is heavy. I guess I wish that, well, I wish that I could close my eyes and rest for an hour and then be able to get up and do what I want. Sometimes I can and sometimes I can't. But it's a heaviness in my body.	*Local Sensation.*
Just use more words for heaviness. Or even an image.	*Urging her to go to Delusion to move the case deeper.*
The image I always used when I was first diagnosed and tried to explain about my legs, was that it was like having five-pound weights attached to my legs, dragging them around. Just dragging. Dragging. Dragging my body around. You know, but now I also lie down because I have to rest my leg. So now one is feeding into the other.	*Local Sensation and Delusion.* *So far we have Fall Back, Gesture, Dragging Weights, Heaviness.....*
Just describe having to drag this five-pound weight around.	
Well, it used to be the left leg, and now the left leg seems to be the stronger leg. And it's probably dragging two legs, but it's definitely dragging this right leg that's in pain most of the	

CASE 2 of WOMAN with MS TEXT of CASE	ANALYSIS of CASE
time. It's just difficult. It's just <u>heavy</u> and <u>doesn't want to move</u>. <u>It just wants to stay stationary</u>.	
So it's heavy and there's dragging. These two. Just, I'm going to keep asking the same questions. You're explaining it very well. It's very clear. It's just, the more it becomes unique to you. . .so more about this heavy and dragging.	*Focusing on these as she keeps repeating them.*
It's just like additional weight that I seem to have to carry. It's the additional weight, this heavy leg that doesn't want to work on its own, that needs a crutch. <u>It</u> needs assistance. <u>It</u> can't do it on its own. It's just this heavy. <u>It's</u> with me all the time and <u>it</u> won't leave me. I don't have <u>it</u> at night and I don't have <u>it</u> in the morning—the pain. <u>It's</u> when I've been on my body. It's maybe my body's way of saying, "slow down," manifesting itself through pain in the leg. But I also have just a fatigue, of <u>just a mind-fog</u> (*New HG*).	*Pattern of Separation coming through with "it". She uses this earlier with her description of the leg as well. This separation hints at Animal Kingdom.* *Delusion plus some Energy with the Gesture. Since there is not much Energy in the case, any Gesture becomes very meaningful.*
A mind-fog, as in?	
Just needing to rest. You know, <u>just like a layer</u>. <u>Like I can't quite see or get out of where I am</u>. <u>It's just this layer of something blocking me, a cloud or something that I can't push through</u>. (*Strong HG showing this layer over her head.*)	*Delusion Level with Gestures and Energy. Beginning to Listen for Kingdom Language as we are moving deeper into the case and Sensation is opening up.*
Very good. Just describe this layer that you can't push through. It can be in the imagination—it doesn't have to make sense.	*Giving the client permission to go into the Unknown. She closes her eyes.....*
<u>It's like a curtain</u>. (*Big HG to indicate.*) A heavy <u>curtain that I want to get by, I want to get out of, get beyond</u>. <u>I want to get beyond this curtain, but I can't</u>. It's just there, and I feel like I can't <u>chip away at it</u>. And <u>that's kind of the fatigue</u>. <u>I want to do these things, but I can't</u>. <u>I can't reach that</u>.	*Delusion Level with Lots of Energy and Gestures. Refers back to the Chief Complaint – good confirmation we are in the right place.*
And chip away means what for you?	*Repeat back her words.*
<u>Break it down</u>. <u>Chip away</u>. <u>Breaking it down</u>. <u>Trying to crawl my way out</u> (*HG*), <u>burrowing my</u>	*Now she gives the Experience of the Delusion and begin to hear Kingdom*

CASE 2 of WOMAN with MS TEXT of CASE	ANALYSIS of CASE
way out of this, getting past this. Ripping it. Anything that will let me escape. I guess escape.	*Language – Animal Kingdom Language. This is confirms the hint we heard earlier of separation "it".*
Just more of this breaking it down, chipping it away, crawl away, burrowing.	*Repeat Back Sensation/Kingdom Language and urge her to go deeper......*
Yes, escaping from this. Getting out of this. This cocoon, I guess. Maybe it's a cocoon feeling, that my body is wrapped and I can't really get out of it. I'm just tightly woven. Tightly woven. (Moves in Chair)	*More Kingdom Language and now Source Language coming through.*
Yes, very good. More of this cocoon feeling, tightly wrapped, tightly woven, whatever comes to mind.	*Repeat Back Kingdom and Source Words.*
I'm picturing a mummy. I'm picturing being wrapped in gauze. My arms and legs and I can't get out. I can't get out, to do what I have to do.	*Delusion and Sensation Language at the Level of Sensation.* *She also refers back to her part of her Chief Complaint of not being able to do what she has to do – this connection assures us we are on solid ground.*
What else do you see with this image? It doesn't have to be about you so much anymore.	*Dissociate the client from herself and have her go deeper into Sensation and Energy Level. Her eyes are closed.*
Well, it's more of a bug. Like probably a caterpillar or a moth, or a butterfly or something. Just a bug. I'm seeing a bug with big eyes.	*Source.........*
A little bit more about this bug with big eyes?	
It's just a bug wrapped in gauze, with big eyes.	
And then what happens to this bug?	
The bug is just there. The bug is just there, trying to squirm. Squirming, trying to get its appendages released. And it can't. The gauze is just too tight. It's wrapped too tight. And it can't. And it's squirming, it's **frustrated, and it can't get out of its own way. And maybe it should stop trying so hard and rest.** Maybe the gauze will not be as hard to release. And I just see it fighting. It's fighting that gauze. It's	*Animal Source Language.* *The Feeling in the Room shifts.........she is in the Energy Level......* *Connects this Source Language with words she used earlier to describe herself.*

CASE 2 of WOMAN with MS TEXT of CASE	ANALYSIS of CASE
fighting to get out. Fighting to get out of that cocoon. And be free.	
And then what happens? It's fighting to get out. . .	*Urges her to go further – listening for anything that doesn't fit.*
It's fighting to get out of the cocoon, and then once it gets out, it's free. But it hasn't gotten out. Once it gets out it would be free.	
If it gets out, what would happen then?	
It will just sail off. Just fly and do whatever it wants to do. Be free.	
What does that look like to be sailing off and flying?	
Beautiful. Free. In the air. Not being weighted down. It can do whatever it wants to do. Just sailing, flying through the air. It grows up. It grew up from being a little bug to being a full butterfly.	*Animal Source Language but listening carefully for anything that doesn't fit.*
And what would that be like then, for this bug?	
A real milestone. To really grow up, take responsibility.	
Anything else you see with this?	
Just very happy, the bug is very happy on its own. Out just circling around, enjoying freedom.	
And you said the other part is that either you push through, or you just, you fall back on it. You either focus, or you fall back on it.	*Going back to the Vital Expression to see if it all comes together.*
Well, sometimes I'm not sure. I use that as an excuse. I'm not sure if I'm resting my leg or if I'm resting because of the fatigue. I sometimes can't distinguish. Sometimes they both come together, and I wonder whether I fall back on that as an excuse.	
And the feeling of when you fall back?	
I guess I don't feel that I'm fighting as much as I	

CASE 2 of WOMAN with MS TEXT of CASE	ANALYSIS of CASE
should be. I'm giving into it. And I should be fighting it. I should be stronger.	
Any more? Should be stronger, should be fighting it. . .	
I guess using it as an excuse. I'm not sure whether I'm, when I say fall back, I'm using it as an excuse for not doing anything. I can say, "well, I'm resting." But I need to rest. And thinking that I need to rest. And wondering if maybe I don't need to, but I've fallen into a pattern.	
So more of this fall, what is falling? If you had to explain it to someone who didn't know English, fallen, falling, fall back. . .	
Umm, reverting to it. Reverting back to a different situation. I might think I need to rest, when actually I don't, but I may not be doing anything. And so I may just, in my own mind, have talked myself into, "This is good, I have to rest. It's okay, I have to rest." I mean, the doctor tells me I have to rest all the time. I'm just used—was used—to being very active. I was used to being quite active and always doing things. And I spend a lot of time by myself. And I sometimes worry about that, that I'm spending too much time under the disguise of "resting." When that's still not very clear sometimes in my mind. I know I need to rest, but. . .	
What's this needing to rest, but. . .	
I sometimes wonder whether I use resting as an excuse to explain not doing something. Not going somewhere, not doing something. And it probably is perfectly legitimate; it might just be in my mind, that I need some kind of validation that this is real, that I have to do this. And I think it's probably because fatigue is so subjective. Nobody feels my fatigue but me. Nobody understands the fatigue. And it's very difficult. You can't see fatigue. You can see that I walk with a cane; you can see that I limp; you can see I	

CASE 2 of WOMAN with MS TEXT of CASE	ANALYSIS of CASE
have a brace—but you can't see fatigue. You can't see the pain in my leg. These are all the invisible symptoms. You can't see the pain in my shoulder. You can see that I can't raise my arm, but you can't see it—it's invisible.	
Talk about this invisible. What does invisible mean?	
It's not outwardly apparent. People can't see it. You talk about it, but it's not something that people can see or feel. They can be tired. "Oh, I was tired when I was pregnant." And it's very difficult to get that across, that when I get fatigue; it's a fatigue that I can't do anything about. So I try to prevent it by resting. And that is, I think, what is tying it, I try to prevent that crash by resting.	
And the crashes, how do you experience the crash?	.
When you hit the wall. Sometimes I've just done way too much and I know I should have rested. But if I didn't have time, then I am just a total zombie. And then I couldn't will anything, my body couldn't do anything. Then I had to rest. And when I worked, I had to lie down everyday at work. I laid down from like 1:00 pm to 2:00 pm. And that was stretching it. It should have been much earlier, but that was the easiest break time. And it was very difficult. It was embarrassing. And people didn't understand. "Oh, Nancy's resting." Well, you know, it was hard. I mean, who rests at work? Well, somebody with a disability rests at work.	
A little more about this total zombie, hit the wall, you can't will yourself. . .	
I just can't function. It's saying, "You've done it, you've got to stop. You can't do one more thing. Stop."	
As if?	
As if someone just put a wall in front of me.	

CASE 2 of WOMAN with MS TEXT of CASE	ANALYSIS of CASE
And it wouldn't let me take one more step. I've just come right up against.	
Can you describe this pain in your right leg, what it's like?	
The pain is, it's just a dull, aching pain on the right side of my leg. It's just dull, achy. Sometimes it travels. At the beginning, it traveled all the way up my leg to my buttocks. And now it's really confined to just to the lower part of my leg, on the side. And usually it's from being on my legs, maybe in one position for too long, or maybe if I'm sitting. I don't have it now, because I've released the brace. And I'm keeping my leg at 90 degrees. But if I was to put my legs up, I would get this pain because I couldn't put my foot into a neutral position. I couldn't find neutral without pain.	
And what does that mean to find neutral?	
To find just a very comfortable position. What I call neutral is the way your foot would usually go. Just the way it would fall. You're lying on the couch, you're reading a book, you don't pay attention to where your feet are. . .but I pay attention. I can't help but pay attention to my right leg, because it doesn't go anywhere right, and it hurts. But if I ice it and put it into this resting splint a coupe of times, I haven't had pain like I have had, so this is working. But they don't know if it will ever go away. I want to do what I did when I was 25.	
What would it be like to do what you did when you were 25?	
No cares, no worries. You did what you wanted; you just did what you wanted. You didn't think about it, you didn't plan your time. You were just free and you did what you wanted. You know, your body behaved. I mean, it wasn't misbehaving. And I didn't think about it. Although I had MS then, too. But I didn't know I had it. I just went and did what I wanted.	

CASE 2 of WOMAN with MS TEXT of CASE	ANALYSIS of CASE
And what is it like to do what you want?	
Oh, lack of responsibility. Not lack of responsibility, but not a heightened sense of responsibility. Young. And you could just do what you wanted to do.	
A little bit more, just in the imagination. What is it like to have this lack of responsibility and just do what you want to do?	
No cares, no worries. No responsibilities. Nobody else to think about. No health issues. No. . . .	
And the experience in the body of that, the sensations in the body?	
I don't know what sensations, but whatever positive. . .just everything working, everything working together. Feeling good. Just feeling good.	
Just describe feeling good more.	
Yes, just an overall sense of well-being.	
So imagine in the body what that would feel like.	
Relaxed. So relaxed. Just relaxed. Comfortable.	
Sensation words for that, comfortable, relaxed. . .	
Energetic. Flexible. Fast. Boundless.	
That's a lot of words. Fast. Flexible. Energetic. Boundless.	
Energetic is the key.	
More words for energetic? It can be in the imagination now, what that would be.	
Happy-go-lucky, just dynamic.	
Great.	
Full of zest. Fun. Fun. Free. Free. Free.	

CASE 2 of WOMAN with MS TEXT of CASE	ANALYSIS of CASE
Any images with this? Energetic, happy-go-lucky. . .	
Yes, just bouncing around. Just skipping rope. Child-like, I suppose.	
Can you describe this pain in the shoulder, what's that like?	
That's an achy, achy, I said achy, limiting. . .a very limiting pain. I mean, I know I can't do certain things or I'll be in severe pain and I risk doing damage to it. I have to have a replacement. I have to have a shoulder replacement, and I'm not doing that until I absolutely have to do it. I'm doing stretching, which has really been helping. I've been going to a really good stretching class. And it's annoying, I can't lift my arm. I can't lift it above here (HG). I can't carry anything. And if I was carrying something, I would pay a price and be sore. But that is not as bad, because I don't walk on it. I mean, this is serious. Probably more serious than my leg, but I don't walk on it. And I have learned to compensate, as I have with most everything with my MS. And I don't use my left hand as much as I should, because that's my weak side anyway. So that was probably the big issue before the leg, but now the leg is certainly much more of a concern.	
What other physical problems do you have?	
Really just MS, the insomnia, and the arthritis in my shoulders.	
So just talk a little bit about the symptoms you have with the MS.	
I have weakness on my left side, going on to my right side now. Weakness. I have foot-drop in both feet now. I have some bladder issues. I have some depression with it.	
And the bladder issues are what?	
Just going to the bathroom too much, needing to go more often. And I have restless leg syndrome on my left leg. My leg jumps all over the place.	

CASE 2 of WOMAN with MS TEXT of CASE	ANALYSIS of CASE
It jumps?	
Yes.	
What happens?	
If I'm lying in bed, it's when I really start to get comfortable, my leg will just start jumping. It just starts moving, my left leg. And it's just unpleasant. And I do take medication, which I'd like to get off. And now that I'm braced on two legs, I'm already seeing some changes in some things in my body.	
What are these?	
Well, I had for years, I had a pain in my left hip/buttocks area. And I've had it off and on for years. And it would just be a sensation, like uncomfortable, and it started to get really bad. It was usually at night when I would lay down, but then it would start to be more often. And then, about a year ago, it started more frequently. And last year when it started, I started to get really dizzy with it. And it would be really unbearable. And Tylenol would work, so my neurologist thought that it was a muscle spasm. So I have been stretching it. But I noticed when I got the new brace, on my left leg, and this toe-op, I haven't had it. So that was good, because that was getting to be so unpleasant. And I would just get so dizzy.	
How would you get dizzy? What was this?	
My head would just start spinning and my eyes would start to feel. . .I would start to feel it in my head before I actually got it. And that was just maybe the last six months. But that's all gone now. Well, knock on wood, I haven't had it. And I'm walking much better in these two braces.	
And how do you experience the insomnia, but now you're taking medications, right. . .	
Well I would be reading or watching TV or	

CASE 2 of WOMAN with MS TEXT of CASE	ANALYSIS of CASE
something and I would be following asleep. And I would get into bed and I would be wide awake. Wide awake. And I would just be up. Or I might fall asleep, but then I would wake up at 2 or 3 in the morning. Now, it started about 20 years ago, I know. And I had gone back to school, so I just assumed, "oh, I must be nervous, I should go study." So I fed into that problem and I would start studying at three, not knowing that this was not a call for studying. And then at that time, my mother also died, and that was hard. So that was when this insomnia started. But I think I always had problems sleeping. Not insomnia. But, I was never a good sleeper. It would be like that I was just awake at night, I would just be there. I might fall asleep, but then I'd wake up early. And then my restless mind. So I would wake up exhausted.	
So the restless mind is what?	
My mind would just go. I would have all this time to think about why I wasn't sleeping and to rehash everything that was going on. And by the time I woke up, I was exhausted.	
And this depression that you experience, how do you experience that?	
Well, it's probably as a result of the MS. But I've just had different bouts of it. And I just was really depressed recently because I need to move and find housing. And it really just rocked my world because I've been paying outrageous rent in the hopes that my place might go condo. So now I am looking for housing, but everything is so expensive. You get nothing for your money here. And I have money, because I've had money for ten years as a deposit. But it buys nothing. And I'm not working now, so my income is less, obviously. So I wouldn't qualify for much of a mortgage, and I'm not sure if I'm going to be able to afford anything here. And I don't think I want to go through this again with renting.	
So how do you experience this then?	

CASE 2 of WOMAN with MS TEXT of CASE	ANALYSIS of CASE
This depression?	
Yes.	
God, this was the worst. I was extremely anxious, which was new for me. I was out of control. I was the worst. It rocked my world. I don't know what it did, but it just made me so insecure. . .so alone. . .so fearful. And it just brought up all issues with family, you know, family issues and everything. And it just was very difficult. I also had questioned whether it was the medication I was on, and I had mentioned that to my doctor a couple of times. I asked to go off of it, and I said, "do you think that could be the cause?" And she said, "well, we'll never know." The next day, the anxiety was gone.	
What was it that you were on?	
Prozac. So, I don't know, but I was on Prozac. And it's very subtle. It was subtle the way it occurred.	
Talk about that, how it occurred.	
It created anxiety and fear in me, but it was so subtle. I can't tell you when. . .I didn't notice it in the beginning, so it must have been very, very subtle, but I new that all of the sudden I was having this fear of driving. And you know, I didn't want to drive. I thought people we're going to hit me. And other fears I had never had before, anxieties. And as soon as I went off it, I thought, "oh my god, I feel good today—I'm so relaxed." It was the Prozac. Umm, out of control, just totally desperate. And I probably blew everything out of proportion. Although it probably wasn't earth-shattering, it became that way for me.	
And earth-shattering means what?	
It just affected everything. I just felt that I had to make some major changes: I couldn't stay; I	

CASE 2 of WOMAN with MS TEXT of CASE	ANALYSIS of CASE
couldn't do this; I couldn't afford it; where was this money going to come from; I was on a fixed income. And I also, when I spoke to the management office, the man was very rude to me, very nasty. And I've been there 30 years. They have helped me, they have, you know, I have a disability. But, there's no protection today for people with disabilities or for the elderly. And my best bet was to go through this guy. But, you know, if he can get a lot more money, and I'm paying good money, but he can get more. And he was as nasty. . .he's a young little thing, you know, who should not be in this job and have this kind of power. And I knew not to take it personally, but it really hit me.	
So, what else physical? Were there other problems?	
During the depression? Oh, I couldn't eat, I couldn't sleep. Even with Ambien I was up. I couldn't eat, I couldn't sleep. I was just playing it over and over again in my mind. Probably so I wouldn't forget it. And you know, the weather was bad, so even if I wanted to, I couldn't get out. It just all fed into itself.	
So of all the physical stuff—the right leg, the shoulder, the weakness, the insomnia, the depression—what else?	
I think we've got it.	Remedy: limenitis bredowii californica Potency: 30C

Overview: Client stuck at fact/name level, denies sensation. Melissa describes levels to urge client deeper. Asks client to describe hand gesture. After getting to source quickly goes back to VE and explores other complaints.

Chief Complaint: severe fatigue and pain with MS

Vital Expression: fall back + HG repeated (first sign of energy in case)

Non Human Specific language homeopath asks about once VE is identified:

Focus and fall back
HG – *what is this?*
HG + focus + will your body – *use more words*
Focus + willing your body
Focus + willing your body + having to do it – *what is sensation? Try to imagine*
More tired – *how do you experience?*
Heaviness – *more words or image*
Having to drag a 5-pound weight - *describe*
Heaviness and dragging – *just these two, more words*
Mind fog – *as in?*
This layer you can't push through – *describe in imagination*
Chip away - *means what for you?*
Breaking it down, chipping it away, crawl away, burrowing - *more*
Cocoon feeling, tightly wrapped, tightly woven – *more, whatever comes to mind*

Kingdom Language:

It's just like additional weight that I seem to have to carry. It's the additional weight, this heavy leg that doesn't want to work on its own, that needs a crutch. It needs assistance. It can't do it on its own. It's just this heavy. It's with me all the time and it won't leave me.
Crawl, burrow, ripping, escape

Source Language:

Maybe it's a cocoon feeling, that my body is wrapped and I can't really get out of it. I'm just tightly woven. . .Well, its more of a bug. Like probably a caterpillar or a moth, or a butterfly or something. Just a bug. I'm seeing a bug with big eyes. . . It will just sail off. Just fly and do whatever it wants to do. . . . It grew up from being a little bug to being a full butterfly.

Energy Language:

The bug is just there, trying to squirm. Squirming, trying to get its appendages released. And it can't. The gauze is just too tight. It's wrapped too tight. And it can't. And it's squirming, it's frustrated, and it can't get out of its own way. And maybe it should stop trying so hard and rest. . . Beautiful. Free. In the air. Not being weighted down. It can do whatever it wants to do. Just sailing, flying through the air.

Miasm: It's annoying. It just really interferes with what I want to do.

Case Management and Outcome:

Client came off all drugs, painkillers. No more pain, no more bladder problems at night. No Ambien to sleep, no restless legs. Now goes out and walks with friends.

H. HOMEWORK

I.   Give five examples from your cases of each of the different types of
        language: name, fact, emotion, delusion, sensation, and energy (if possible),
        which could come at any of the different levels.

II.   Extract out of your cases an example of each of the levels: Name, Fact,
        Emotion, Delusion, Sensation and Energy.

III.   Chart one of your cases and give an indication and examples from the case of
        the different levels that you saw in the case. For example, at Level 1, the
        patient says her chief complaint is arthritis; at level 2, the patient says there is
        cramping, >walking, etc.

IV.   What are the difficulties you have encountered trying to apply the levels in
        casetaking? Please explain.

For feedback you can send your homework to Melissa Burch at melissa@innerhealth.us.

About Melissa Burch, CCH

Melissa Burch, CCH, co-founded The Catalyst School of Homeopathy with Christopher Beaver, CCH. She established live phone case supervision and clinics based on the Sensation Method.

She created a unique homeopathic phone referral service with a homeopath team approach. She is president of Inner Health, Inc., which produces numerous online and onsite courses for homeopaths, homeopathic patients and people interested in alternative medicine. She produced the first Radio Series on Homeopathy.

She was the Master Homeopath for the proving of Stoichactis Kenti Sea Anemone. She co-wrote and published the five part "Vital Sensation Manual." Ms. Burch worked with Dr. Nandita Shah at Quiet Healing Center in South India for over a year and half. She graduated from the School of Homeopathy New York, directed by Jo Daly, and the New York School of Homeopathy, directed by Robert Stewart.

About Inner Health, Inc.

Inner Health (IH) provides homeopathic services to the general public and to the homeopathic community. IH is a leader in establishing the highest quality of services in the complementary and alternative medical field through its education, practitioners, workshops and services.

IH's vision is to make homeopathy a household word. Our goal is to identify IH in the consumer's mind as the place to go for the best, natural deep healing on all level—mental, emotional, physical and spiritual; and to create a demand for homeopathy and in particular for Certified IH Homeopaths, through our innovative, educational and creative marketing materials.

Training

IH provides basic and post-graduate training for homeopaths to develop reliable and better results in their practices by following the IH Approach—a systematic way of case taking and analysis based on the Sensation Method—and by implementing the IH System, which includes case management protocols, scripts and information, client business services and marketing.

Homeopaths have the opportunity to train and become Certified IH Homeopaths through workshops, supervision and educational materials. Combined with our own extensive marketing of IH and the IH approach to homeopathy, which results in constant referrals to Certified IH Homeopaths, IH Homeopaths will have a unique and wonderful opportunity to develop themselves as professional homeopaths, heal others, share clinical information with the homeopathic community, be well paid and have excellent systems to guide them to provide the highest care to the client.

Printed in Great Britain
by Amazon